CORONARY
HEART DISEASE

Contemporary Patient Management Series

- *Acute Renal Failure,* Edward Kuehnel, M.D., and William Bennett, M.D.

- *Bleeding Disorders,* Jessica H. Lewis, M.D., Joel A. Spero, M.D., and Ute Hasiba, M.D.

- *Stroke,* Lowell G. Lubic, M.D., and Harry P. Palkovitz, M.D.

- *Tuberculosis,* Douglas R. Gracey, M.D., and Whitney W. Addington, M.D.

- *Chronic Obstructive Pulmonary Disease,* Warren C. Miller, M.D.

- *Renal Tubular Dysfunction,* Vardaman M. Buckalew, Jr., M.D., and Michael A. Moore, M.D.

- *Infections in Obstetrics and Gynecology,* Lester T. Hibbard, M.D.

- *Pain: Origin and Treatment,* Benjamin H. Gorsky, M.D.

- *Rheumatoid Arthritis,* edited by Duncan A. Gordon, M.D.

- *Chronic Duodenal Ulcer,* G. Gordon McHardy, M.D.

- *Anxiety: A Guide to Biobehavioral Diagnosis and Therapy for Physicians and Mental Health Clinicians,* Richard J. Goldberg, M.D.

- *Inflammatory Bowel Disease,* Marshall Sparberg, M.D.

- *Headache,* Seymour Diamond, M.D., and Arnold P. Friedman, M.D.

- *Osteoarthritis and Musculoskeletal Pain Syndromes,* edited by Bernard F. Germain, M.D.

- *Peptic Ulcer,* Herman J. Kaplan, M.D.

- *Sexually Transmitted Diseases: Guide to Diagnosis and Therapy,* Third Edition, Robert C. Noble, M.D.

- *Coronary Heart Disease,* Robert M. Davidson, M.D.

CORONARY HEART DISEASE

Robert M. Davidson, M.D.,
F.A.C.P., F.A.C.C.
Associate Clinical Professor of Medicine
University of California, Los Angeles,
School of Medicine
Attending Cardiologist
Cedars-Sinai Medical Center
and UCLA Medical Center
Los Angeles, California

MEDICAL EXAMINATION PUBLISHING CO., INC.
an Excerpta Medica company

Davidson, Robert M. (Robert Martin), (date)
   Coronary heart disease.

   (Contemporary patient management series)
   Bibliography: p.
   Includes index.
   1. Coronary heart disease. I. Title. II. Series.
[DNLM: 1. Coronary Disease. WG 300 D253c]
RC685.C6D38   1984   616.1'23   84-18993
ISBN 0-87488-874-3

Printed in the United States of America

This book is dedicated to the memory of my parents, Lillian and Nathaniel, and to my wife Susan, and children Hillary and Michael for their patience, understanding, and invaluable help.

Contents

Preface

Coronary artery disease remains the single largest cause of death among adults in the United States. As a result of recent advances in diagnosis and treatment and attention to preventative measures, the death rate has been declining in the last 15 years. The first section of this book deals with the diagnosis of coronary heart disease, and the remaining sections with its treatment, including a chapter on primary and secondary prevention, a subject in which some recent discoveries may have major impact. In the last chapter, some typical clinical case examples are presented and discussed to illustrate the clinical application of the principles presented throughout the text.

The clinical spectrum of coronary artery disease ranges from the individual with undetected asymptomatic coronary disease to the patient who has had multiple myocardial infarctions and severe heart failure. In between these extremes lie the majority of patients who come to our attention, including the minimally symptomatic patients, the symptomatic patients with chronic angina pectoris, and the patients presenting with acute myocardial infarction. In many cases, each of these examples represents a stage in the slow and gradual progression of the disease, while in others, the disease may present dramatically, and all too often, fatally. It is the unpredictability of this disease that makes its treatment often uncertain and challenging. Although there is often a lack of agreement among experts as to the correct approach to certain aspects of this disease, the aim of this book is to present the most generally agreed upon approaches, along with a discussion of alternative concepts of diagnosis and treatment.

Acknowledgments

A number of people deserve credit for their assistance in the preparation of this book. I am indebted to Joy Nunn, Barbara Voight and Dolores Lawry for their multiple hours spent in typing and word processing and to Patty Edwards, Cassie Evans, Lance Laforteza and Portia Simmons for their help in preparation of the illustrations. I owe thanks to Marcia Wallis for her secretarial assistance.

I also wish to thank Drs. Daniel Berman and William Ganz for their advice and contributions.

Finally, I am especially indebted to the family and friends of the late Dr. Ferenc Solti, whose kind contributions in his memory made this effort possible.

notice

The author and the publisher of this book have made every effort to ensure that all therapeutic modalities that are recommended are in accordance with accepted standards at the time of publication.

The drugs specified within this book may not have specific approval by the Food and Drug Administration in regard to the indications and dosages that are recommended by the author. The manufacturer's package insert is the best source of current prescribing information.

Chapter 1

DIAGNOSIS OF CORONARY ARTERY DISEASE IN THE ASYMPTOMATIC PATIENT

It is the asymptomatic patient with coronary artery disease who represents the greatest challenge to detection and treatment. Although only a small proportion of the general adult population has asymptomatic, but significant coronary artery disease, it is precisely this group that must be identified and treated if we are to make a meaningful impact on morbidity and mortality in this disease. In many patients, however, transition from asymptomatic to symptomatic is sudden and dramatic, often presenting with severe myocardial infarction or fatal ventricular fibrillation.

Since the asymptomatic patient is, by definition, free of complaints, he generally does not seek medical attention and will therefore remain undiagnosed. Fortunately, however, many of these patients come to our attention as part of a routine general checkup, or for an unrelated complaint. Since the routine history, physical examination, chest x-ray, laboratory data, and even the electrocardiogram fail to detect asymptomatic coronary artery disease in the vast majority of cases, we must rely upon other means for detection of "silent" coronary artery disease.

RISK FACTORS

The identification of risk factors for coronary disease in a given individual is an important initial step in the screening of asymptomatic individuals. Important risk factors include age (55 or greater), male sex, positive family history of coronary disease, hypertension, hypercholesterolemia, smoking, diabetes mellitus, and obesity.

EXERCISE STRESS TESTING

Although it has recently been emphasized that routine electrocardiographic stress testing of asymptomatic individuals is not very cost-effective because of the relatively low predictive value of this test in this population, it still remains our most effective diagnostic tool in this disease, particularly when applied to those subjects with one or more risk factors. Since the likelihood of existence of coronary artery disease increases as the number of risk factors increases in any given individual, the indication for exercise stress testing in an asymptomatic individual increases with the number of positive risk factors. There is probably little justification for performing a stress test in the absence of one or more risk factors.

NEGATIVE STRESS TEST

If the exercise stress test is negative in all respects (absence of symptoms, normal heart rate and blood pressure response, normal duration of exercise, and normal electrocardiographic response) (see Chapter 3), the likelihood of significant coronary artery disease in such an individual is very low, and no further workup is indicated. The exercise test should be repeated at intervals according to the patient's age and number of risk factors, usually varying from 1 to 3 years.

POSITIVE STRESS TEST

As is discussed in further detail in Chapter 3, a number of criteria are considered in the classification of an exercise stress test as "positive" or "negative." Included in these criteria for an abnormal, or "positive" test are significant ST segment depression on the electrocardiogram, failure to exercise more than 6 minutes (Stage 2 of the Bruce Protocol), failure to achieve 90% of the age-predicted heart rate, and the development of chest pain during exercise. Using these criteria, a positive exercise stress test in an asymptomatic individual is still not necessarily indicative of coronary artery disease, and the physician's response to a positive test in such an individual should depend upon the specifics of the test results as well as upon the clinical setting. In a recent study (Hopkirk et al.), the combination of the presence of at least one clinical risk factor combined with: (1) development of at least 0.3 mV horizontal or downsloping ST segment depression which begins by Stage II, (2) persistence of at least 0.1 mV ST depression for at least 6 minutes into recovery, and (3) total exercise duration of less than 10 minutes, had a predictive value of 85% for two- and three-vessel coronary artery disease (although only a 33% sensitivity). The primary goal of exercise testing in asymptomatic individuals should be to identify those individuals with multivessel or left main coronary disease, who are at high risk for subsequent cardiac events. Thus, a highly positive test in a healthy young individual with a number of risk factors should generally lead to a different course of action than a mildly positive test in an older individual who also has many other physical problems.

In many cases, "asymptomatic" individuals are asymptomatic because they do not exercise sufficiently in their routine activities to provoke symptoms of angina pectoris. In these cases, exercise stress tests can provoke typical anginal pectoris as well as showing other indications of the presence of coronary artery disease. In such an individual, the combination of the development of symptoms in the presence of other indications of positivity on the stress test establishes the diagnosis of coronary artery disease with a fair amount of certainty. Other individuals with coronary artery disease are truly asymptomatic even under conditions in which they develop myocardial ischemia and thus remain asymptomatic while performing an exercise stress test which shows electrocardiographic changes consistent with ischemia.

Since the incidence of false-positive stress tests in the asymptomatic population is high, it is usually desirable to perform a confirmatory test in these individuals such as a thallium stress test, exercise wall motion test, or coronary fluoroscopy (see Chapters 4 and 5). In certain cases it is desirable to go directly from a positive exercise stress test to coronary arteriography, such as when the test is highly positive in all respects (and critical coronary artery disease is therefore suspected) or when the correct diagnosis is essential. The choice of which of these secondary tests to perform in the presence of a positive stress test depends upon the availability of the test, the willingness of the patient to undergo further testing, economical considerations, and most important, the question of how the test results will affect decisions in patient management. In general, the thallium stress test, often combined with coronary fluoroscopy, is usually the most useful test in the further assessment of an asymptomatic positive exercise stress test. If the thallium stress test is negative, and particularly if both thallium test and coronary fluoroscopy are negative, the likelihood is that the electrocardiographic stress test is a false-positive one, and that no significant coronary artery disease is present. On the other hand, a positive thallium test combined with evidence of calcium within one or more coronary arteries on coronary fluoroscopy in conjunction with a positive exercise stress test is almost always indicative of significant coronary artery disease.

MANAGEMENT

Having identified the asymptomatic patient with probable coronary artery disease by stress testing, the decisions regarding further management are still controversial. One must be prepared to deal with the implications of asymptomatic coronary artery disease; otherwise, there is no point in performing stress tests on these individuals. One of the main objectives of identifying such patients should be to try to identify those individuals at high risk for sudden death or extensive myocardial infarction. At the present time, such patients will usually be considered for "prophylactic" coronary artery bypass surgery. This decision is based largely upon the coronary anatomy as determined by coronary arteriography. The indications for coronary arteriography in the asymptomatic patient would, in general, be the suspicion of severe coronary artery disease (left main coronary disease or triple-vessel disease) or the necessity of making a definitive diagnosis and determination of the extent of disease in such individuals in whom this would be important (for example: pilots, policemen, firemen, individuals whose lives involve heavy physical work, or individuals whose decisions regarding future plans might be affected by this knowledge). The indicators of severe coronary artery disease (prior to coronary arteriography) would in general include evidence of extensive thallium perfusion defects (see Chapter 4) as well as a high degree of positivity of the various parameters in the electrocardiographic stress test (see Chapter 3).

In patients with positive noninvasive tests who would not be immediately considered for coronary arteriography and coronary bypass surgery because of evidence of limited or single-vessel disease or because of complicating medical or other factors, identification of probable coronary artery disease by stress testing would still be of value in that these patients would then be followed more closely and would be advised to reduce or eliminate factors which might increase their risks (see Chapter 11). Although the management of the asymptomatic patient with coronary artery disease remains controversial, a general scheme for diagnosis and management of these individuals is given in Figure 1-1.

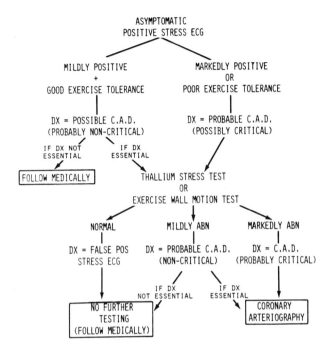

Figure 1-1. A flow chart for the management of the patient with an asymptomatic stress ECG. See text for discussion. (DX = Diagnosis, C.A.D. = Coronary Artery Disease, Pos = Positive, ABN = Abnormal, ECG = Electrocardiogram)

REFERENCES

Bruce, R. A. , Hossack, K. F. , DeRouen, T. A. , and Hofer, V. : Enhanced risk assessment for primary coronary heart disease events by maximal exercise testing: 10 years' experience of Seattle Heart Watch. J Am Coll Cardiol 2, 1983, pp. 565-573.

Cohn, P. F. : Asymptomatic coronary artery disease, pathophysiology, diagnosis, management. Mod Concepts Cardiovasc Dis 50, 1981, pp. 55-60.

Cohn, P. F. : Prognosis and treatment of asymptomatic coronary artery disease. J Am Coll Cardiol 1, 1983, pp. 959-964.

Ellestad, M. H. : "Stress Testing," Ed. 2, F. A. Davis Co. , Philadelphia, 1980, pp. 377-384.

Giagnoni, E. , Secchi, M. B. , Wu, S. C. , Morabito, A. ,
Oltrona, L. , Mancarella, S. , Volpin, N. , Fossa, L. ,
Bettazzi, L. , Arangio, G. , Sachero, A. , and Folli, G. :
Prognostic value of exercise EKG testing in asymptomatic
normotensive subjects. N Engl J Med 309, 1983, pp. 1085-
1089.

Hopkirk, J. A. C. , Uhl, G. S. , Hickman, T. R. Jr. , Fischer,
T. , and Medina, A. : Discriminant value of clinical and exercise variables in detecting significant coronary artery disease
in asymptomatic men. J Am Coll Cardiol 3, 1984, pp. 887-894.

Iskandrian, A. S. , Segal, B. L. , and Anderson, G. S. : Asymptomatic myocardial ischemia. Arch Int Med 141, 1981, pp. 95-
97.

Kent, K. M. , Rosing, D. R. , Ewels, C. J. , Lipson, L. ,
Bonow, R. , and Epstein, S. E. : Prognosis of asymptomatic or
mildly symptomatic patients with coronary artery disease. Am
J Cardiol 49, 1982, pp. 1823-1831.

Chapter 2

DIAGNOSIS OF CORONARY ARTERY DISEASE IN THE SYMPTOMATIC PATIENT

In one sense, the diagnosis of coronary artery disease is great-ly facilitated by a history of chest pain compared to the individ-ual just considered in the first chapter with asymptomatic disease; but in another sense, the patient presenting with a history of chest pain represents a challenge in diagnosis, since there is a multitude of causes of chest pain other than coronary artery disease (Table 2-1). Fortunately, the characteristic symptom pattern of "typical" angina pectoris is so distinctive that when such a history is obtained, the diagnosis of coronary artery disease is almost certain.

HISTORY

TYPICAL ANGINA PECTORIS

In "classic" angina pectoris, the patient experiences a sensa-tion of pressure or heaviness in the midchest area, precipitated by physical or emotional stress which is relieved within min-utes by rest or elimination of the stress. Exposure to cold temperatures may precipitate angina or lower the threshold for it. The discomfort often (but not always) radiates beyond the chest to the throat, jaw, shoulder(s), arm(s), and/or back. Typically, the pain is not affected by movement, position, or breathing, and there is no associated tenderness of the chest wall. A simple and useful test to distinguish the pain of angina pectoris from noncardiac pain is the administration of a sub-lingual tablet of nitroglycerin to a patient during an episode of pain. The pain due to angina pectoris is usually relieved within a minute of taking the nitroglycerin, while noncardiac pain (with the possible exception of esophageal spasm) is not affected by nitroglycerin. Failure of nitroglycerin to relieve cardiac pain may also result from stale (old) tablets or because the chest pain is due to sustained coronary insufficiency or acute myocardial infarction rather than to a simple episode of angina pectoris.

7

Table 2-1.   Common Causes of Chest Pain

I. Cardiac
    A. Coronary Artery Disease
        1. Angina Pectoris
            a. Typical
            b. Atypical
            c. Resting
            d. Variant
        2. Acute Myocardial Infarction
    B. Valvular Disease
        1. Aortic Stenosis
        2. Mitral Valve Prolapse
    C. Myocardial Disease
        1. Acute Myocarditis
        2. Hypertrophic Cardiomyopathy (I. H. S. S.)
        3. "Syndrome X" (Angina pectoris with normal coronary arteries)
    D. Pericardial Disease
        1. Acute Pericarditis
        2. Dressler's Syndrome

II. Vascular
    A. Dissecting Aortic Aneurysm
    B. Pulmonary Hypertension
    C. Pulmonary Embolism

III. Thoracic
    A. Pneumothorax
    B. Pleurisy
    C. Thoracic Outlet Syndrome

IV. Musculoskeletal
    A. Costochondritis (Tietze's Syndrome)
    B. Cervical Root Syndrome
    C. Chest Wall Trauma
    D. Herpes Zoster

V. Gastrointestinal
    A. Esophageal Spasm
    B. Gastroesophageal Reflux
    C. Esophageal Rupture
    D. Peptic Ulcer
    E. Cholecystitis

"ATYPICAL" ANGINA PECTORIS

Unfortunately (from a diagnostic standpoint), angina pectoris is often "atypical," leading to problems in diagnosis. "Atypical" can refer to the location, character, duration, provocation, or radiation of pain, or even to the absence of pain. Locations of pain other than the chest most often include the same areas to which typical angina pectoris radiates (throat, jaw, teeth, head, neck, back, shoulders, arms, hands, and upper abdomen). It is not uncommon for patients to initially seek care from specialists in areas relating to the site of their pain such as dentists, ear, nose, and throat physicians, orthopedic surgeons, or gastroenterologists. In such cases, where the location is atypical, the tip-off as to the true cause of the pain is usually the history of provocation by physical or emotional stress. Often the sensation is not perceived as pain, and the patient may deny pain but admit to another sensation such as pressure or heaviness, numbness, tingling, burning, or just a vague discomfort. Again, the keys to a correct diagnosis are the precipitation by stress, the brief duration, and the relief by rest, relaxation, or nitroglycerin.

In some cases, the quality and location of the pain or discomfort may be of typical angina pectoris, but there might not be history of preceding exertion or stress, particularly in elderly or debilitated persons whose physical activities may be quite limited. Anginal pain may be brought on by eating ("postprandial angina"), or may occur at rest ("rest angina" or "angina decubitus") or even during sleep ("nocturnal angina"). Angina due to coronary spasm ("Prinzmetal's angina" or "variant angina") typically occurs independent of exertion or stress, and is diagnosed by pain typical of angina in quality and location, in association with characteristic electrocardiographic changes (Figure 2-1).

Whereas typical angina pectoris can usually be diagnosed by the history alone, the diagnosis of atypical angina pectoris almost always needs additional diagnostic tests.

PHYSICAL EXAMINATION

In comparison to the history and to ancillary findings, the physical examination is relatively unrevealing in the diagnosis of coronary artery disease. In fact, there are no findings on physical examinations which are pathognomonic for coronary artery disease. There are, however, certain associated findings which should arouse suspicion of coronary artery disease, such as evidence of the presence of risk factors of coronary disease,

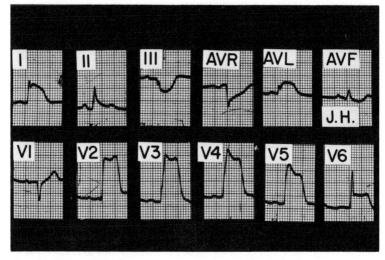

Figure 2-1.   ECG taken during an episode of chest pain in a
patient with prinzmetal's (variant) angina.   The degree of ST
segment elevation in the anterolateral leads (1, A_{VL}, V_2-V_6)
is extreme.

including hypertension, obesity, xanthelasmas and xanthomas,
and diagonal ear lobe creases.   Evidence of peripheral vascular
disease on examination also suggests the coexistence of coronary
disease.   The only cardiac finding that is somewhat suggestive
of coronary artery disease is an early diastolic (S4) gallop (an
indication of decreased left ventricular compliance), which is
helpful in the diagnosis if it is present, but its absence does not
imply the absence of coronary artery disease.   An S4 gallop is
also frequent in hypertension, with or withour coronary artery
disease, as well as other forms of heart disease.   Signs of
congestive heart failure (elevated venous pressure, pulmonary
rales, or S3 gallop or edema) are usually late findings in coronary artery disease, resulting from one or more myocardial
infarctions, and should not be expected in early cases of coronary disease.   Similarly, arrhythmias are usually found later
in the course of coronary artery disease and are very nonspecific
as well.

LABORATORY

Routine laboratory tests are of no value in the diagnosis of coronary artery disease, but the finding of hypercholesterolemia or

elevated blood sugar may indicate predisposing risk factors for coronary disease. Laboratory and x-ray studies may be very helpful in the diagnosis of noncardiac conditions causing chest pain (Table 2-1).

ELECTROCARDIOGRAM

In the absence of previous myocardial infarction, the resting electrocardiogram is not a very sensitive or specific test for coronary artery disease unless it is taken at the time of chest pain. The transient development of ST segment depression of 1 or more millimeters (horizontal or downsloping) during an episode of chest pain with a previously normal ST segment is virtually diagnostic for ischemia and the presence of coronary artery disease (Figure 2-2). Although less specific, the development of new T wave changes (normal to inverted, or inverted to normal) or "nondiagnostic" ST segment changes should also be considered highly suspicious for the presence of coronary artery disease. In variant (Prinzmetal's) angina, transient ST segment elevation (Figure 2-1) rather than ST segment depression is characteristic during pain and is often accompanied by arrhythmias. It is important to bear in mind that a normal electrocardiogram during an episode of chest pain does not rule out the presence of angina pectoris and coronary artery disease but does suggest the possibility of a diagnosis other than coronary artery disease.

COMBINATION OF CLINICAL INFORMATION

Using a clinical profile alone, a reasonably accurate estimate of the presence or absence of significant coronary artery disease may be made in a patient with chest pains prior to performing any confirmatory tests. The single most important piece of information is the type of pain (typical, atypical, or clearly non-anginal). Next in importance in diagnostic value is a history and/or electrocardiographic evidence of prior myocardial infarction. Other clinical data found to be important in a recent study (Pryor et al.) included (in decreasing order) sex (male < female), age, history of smoking, hyperlipidemia, ST-T wave changes in the resting ECG, and the presence of diabetes mellitus.

THE USE OF CONFIRMATORY TESTS

The application of ECG stress tests, nuclear and other non-invasive tests, and coronary arteriography in the diagnosis and characterization of coronary artery disease is discussed in the next four chapters.

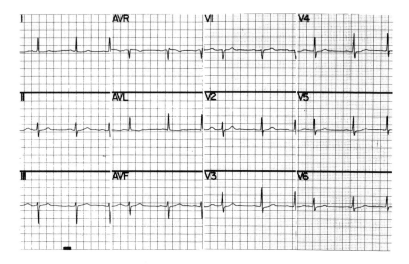

Figure 2-2A.   Three consecutive electrocardiograms taken before (A), during (B), and following (C) an episode of chest pain. In (A) and (C), these are mild nonspecific ST and T wave abnormalities, while in (B) these are marked ST-T changes consistent with ischemia.

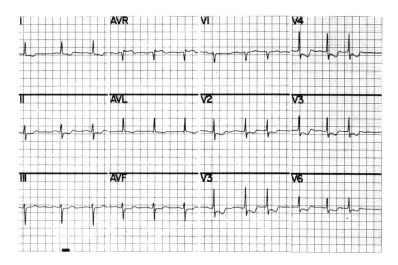

Figure 2-2B.

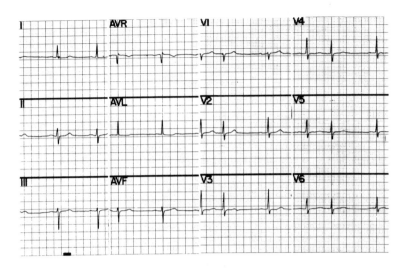

Figure 2-2C.

REFERENCES

Andrus, E. C., and Baker, B. M.: Diagnosis of Angina Pectoris, in "Symposium on Coronary Heart Disease," 2nd Ed., American Heart Association, Inc., New York, 1968, pp. 44-48.

Christie, L. G., and Conti, C. R.: Systematic approach to evaluation of angina-like chest pain: pathophysiology and clinical testing with emphasis on objective documentation of myocardial ischemia. Am Heart J 102, 1981, pp. 897-912.

Hurst, J. W., King, S. B., Walter, P. F., Friesinger, G. C., and Edwards, J. E.: Atherosclerotic coronary heart disease: Angina pectoris, myocardial infarction, and other manifestations of myocardial ischemia, in Hurst, J. W., "The Heart" McGraw-Hill Book Company, New York, 1982, pp. 1020-1058.

Pryor, D. B., Harrell, F. E. Jr., Lee, K. L., Califf, R. M., and Rosati, R. A.: Estimating the likelihood of significant coronary artery disease. Am J Med 75, 1983, pp. 771-780.

Chapter 3

EXERCISE STRESS TESTS

The single most useful and easily administered test for the diagnosis of coronary artery disease is the stress test. Although there are a variety of stress tests available, including the step test (Master's and double Master's), treadmill, and bicycle ergometer, the most commonly employed test at the present time is the treadmill stress test.

INDICATIONS FOR STRESS TESTING

1. Detection of coronary artery disease
2. Confirmation of coronary artery disease
3. Determination of extent and severity of coronary artery disease
4. Evaluation of response to therapy
5. Establishing functional capacity
6. As an indicator of prognosis after acute myocardial infarction
7. To evaluate arrhythmias

CONTRAINDICATIONS TO STRESS TESTING

1. Unstable angina pectoris
2. Recent myocardial infarction (except for low level stress test)
3. Severe hypertension
4. Significant aortic stenosis or severe mitral stenosis
5. Significant congestive heart failure
6. Significant arrhythmias or conduction defects
7. Significant electrolyte abnormalities
8. Significant other illnesses (arthritic diseases, recent injuries, or conditions which would be exacerbated by exercise testing)

FACTORS WHICH MAY INTERFERE WITH
INTERPRETATION OF STRESS TEST

1. Inability to exercise adequately
2. Postprandial state
3. Baseline ST segment abnormalities
4. Atrial fibrillation
5. Left or right bundle branch block
6. Left ventricular hypertrophy
7. Hypokalemia
8. Digitalis
9. Quinidine-type drugs
10. Beta-blocking drugs
11. Tricyclic antidepressant drugs
12. Permanent pacemaker
13. Noncoronary forms of heart disease (cardiomyopathy, valvular diseases (including mitral valve prolapse), congenital heart disease, Wolff-Parkinson-White syndrome)
14. Female sex

PREPARING A PATIENT FOR
EXERCISE STRESS TESTING

The preparation of a patient for exercise stress testing depends to a certain extent upon the type of test to be done as well as the purpose for which the test is being done. For an elective diagnostic stress test, the patient should be in a condition to exercise to his best capability, should not have eaten for several hours, and should be off all medications which will interfere with the interpretation of the test, if at all possible (digitalis drugs can cause a false-positive test and should be discontinued 10-14 days prior to the test, while beta-blocking drugs can blunt the heart rate and blood pressure response and should be discontinued for 36 hours prior to the test). The decision to discontinue medications, particularly digitalis and beta-blocking drugs, must be on an individual basis, since the risk of discontinuing essential medication must be considered compared to the value of the exercise test itself. When beta-blocking drugs are discontinued, this should generally be done on a gradual basis. In some instances it may not be necessary to discontinue these medications: for example, a negative test in the presence of digitalis is still interpretable, as is a positive test on a beta-blocker. At times, it may even be desirable to continue certain medications if part of the reason for performing the test is to evaluate the patient's response to these medications.

Patients should be psychologically as well as physically prepared to take the test, and it is customary to have the patient sign an informed consent form, since there is a small but definite risk to exercise stress testing (serious arrhythmias, provocation of coronary artery insufficiency or acute myocardial infarction, and very rarely, death). An example of an informed consent form is shown in Figure 3-1.

EQUIPMENT AND PERSONNEL REQUIREMENTS

The variety of equipment available today for stress testing is both extensive and expensive, but an elaborate setup is not required. Although such features as automatic programming, computer assisted interpretation, and multichannel monitors and recorders all have their merit, an adequate stress test can be done with a standard motorized treadmill, in which speed and/or elevation can be controlled, or a simple mechanical bicycle ergometer, as well as a single channel electrocardiographic monitor and recorder.

TREADMILL STRESS TEST

Equipment

A motorized treadmill, electrocardiographic monitor, electrocardiographic recorder, disposable ECG electrodes, blood pressure apparatus, defibrillator, oxygen tank and mask, and emergency medication (atropine and lidocaine).

Personnel

Nurse or technician and physician or physician's assistant. A physician should always be immediately available.

BICYCLE STRESS TEST

Equipment and Personnel

The same as for a treadmill test except a bicycle ergometer is used in place of the treadmill.

STEP TEST

Equipment

All that is needed is a set of steps, and a 12-lead electrocardiogram machine.

CONSENT FOR TREADMILL STRESS TESTING

In order to evaluate the ability of my heart to respond to exercise, I voluntarily agree to undergo an exercise stress test in the offices of Dr. _____. The test will be conducted by experienced personnel under the supervision of Dr. _____ _____ and will be carefully monitored.

I understand that this test may in some cases cause symptoms such as palpitations, chest pain, shortness of breath or dizziness, and in very rare cases may even result in fainting, seriously abnormal heart rhythms, and even heart attacks.

I understand that the test may be terminated at any time at my request or when in the determination of Dr. _____, if there is any medical indication to do so.

I have read the above and give my consent to proceed with the test and will not hold the doctors or personnel involved responsible if untoward events or injury results.

Signed: _____

Time: _____
Date: _____
Witness: _____

Figure 3-1. An example of an informed consent form for an exercise stress test.

Personnel

A nurse or technician; a physician should be available but not necessarily directly present.

ELECTRODE APPLICATION AND LEAD SYSTEMS

Although techniques differ between physicians involved in exercise testing, certain principles of electrode placement are essential: (1) the electrodes must be of high quality (preferably silver-silver chloride) to achieve the highest electrical conductance from the skin surface; (2) the adhesive electrode pads must be adequate to keep the electrodes in place throughout the procedure, especially in diaphoretic patients; (3) the skin site must be prepared so that there is a minimum of electrical resistance between the electrode and the skin. For this purpose

appropriate portions of the patient's chest are shaved, if necessary, to remove any hair at the site of electrode application;
(4) the top layer of epidermis is abraded at each site and surface oil is removed by vigorous rubbing of a gauze pad moistened with alcohol, acetone, or ether until the skin site is red. Only after this is done and the skin is dry, should the electrodes be applied. The electrodes should be applied over bones (ribs, clavicles, or sternum) rather than on muscle or fat whenever possible.

Although simultaneous monitoring of several leads is desirable for maximum sensitivity, a single-lead system is sufficient, in which case the lead should be V_5 or a bipolar V_5. Depending upon the equipment available, anything from a single-lead, three-electrode system to a 12-lead, ten-electrode system can be used. A single-lead, V_5-type system will pick up the vast majority of diagnostic ECG changes, while a 3-lead system will detect almost all of the rest of the potential abnormalities which would be detected by a 12-lead system. In a 3-lead system, in addition to the V_5 lead, an inferior and an anterior lead is also obtained. Figure 3-2 illustrates one lead system. In this system the electrode connected to the right arm lead is applied either to the manubrium sternum (CM_5 system) or just below the right clavicle (CS_5 system). The electrode connected to the left arm lead is applied to the V_5 chest position so that when lead 1 is selected on the ECG machine a bipolar V_5 lead results. An electrode is applied to the V_1 or V_2 position and connected to the chest lead on the ECG monitor and recorder, which will result in an anterior lead being recorded. The right leg electrode is applied over the right iliac crest and the left leg electrode over the left iliac crest so that selection of lead 2 on the electrocardiogram results in an inferior lead.

All of the lead wires are secured to the chest with tape so that there is a minimum of movement and stress during the test. In a woman, a brassiere should be worn to minimize movement of the breasts on the chest wall.

Prior to exercise, a 12-lead electrocardiogram should always be obtained as well as a series of tracings from the monitor leads done in the standing and supine positions as well as during hyperventilation and Valsalva maneuvers. The latter is done to establish any "artifactual" changes in ST segments caused by these responses and to distinguish these potential false-positive responses from true ischemic changes after exercise. Blood pressure should be taken prior to exercise in the supine and standing positions as well.

During exercise, the cardiac monitor must be watched continually for changes in heart rate and rhythm and for development

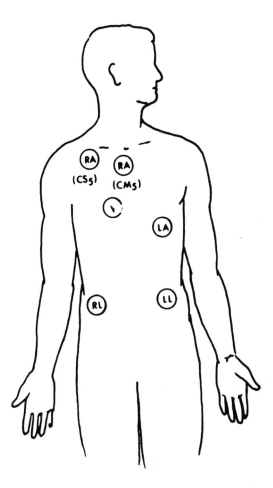

Figure 3-2. The location for electrode placement for a stress test using 5 electrodes. The R. A. electrode is placed in the right infraclavicular area for a bipolar CS_5 lead, or on the manubrium sternum for a bipolar CM_5 lead. The V electrode is in the V_1 position, and the L. A. electrode is in the V_5 position. The R. L. and L. L. electrodes are placed over the right and left iliac crests, respectively.

of ST segment changes. A short ECG strip (at least the V_5 lead and preferably inferior and anterior leads as well) should be recorded every minute during exercise and immediately after cessation of exercise (in both the standing and supine positions) as well as every 2 minutes after cessation of exercise (in the supine position) until 8 minutes is reached or ST segments return to baseline.

EXERCISE PROTOCOLS

TREADMILL TESTS

A variety of test protocols are in common use (Figure 3-3). Some physicians prefer submaximal stress tests, while others prefer maximal stress tests. In the submaximal test, exercise is terminated when the patient reaches 85-90% of his age-predicted maximum heart rate (Table 3-1). In the maximal stress test, the test is terminated when the patient can no longer exercise because of fatigue or other symptoms or when the patient reaches his maximum predicted heart rate. Although the sensitivity of detecting ischemic heart disease is slightly higher in the maximal as opposed to submaximal stress test, this difference is probably small, and the submaximal test is sufficient in most cases to detect coronary artery disease, especially when additional criteria beyond the ECG response are utilized. A number of protocols have been developed for exercise stress testing, all of which share the principle of gradual increase in exercise level. In some protocols, the speed of the treadmill remains constant while the incline is increased every few minutes; in other protocols the incline is maintained constant while the speed is gradually increased in a stepwise fashion. In other protocols, such as the Bruce protocol (Table 3-2), both the speed and inclination are increased stepwise. For individual patients with specific physical problems it may be necessary to modify any given protocol to accommodate the patient.

BICYCLE ERGOMETRY

The principle is the same as in treadmill testing, i.e., there is a stepwise increase in exercise level, accomplished with the bicycle by increasing the resistance to pedaling while the speed is maintained constant. In any of the protocols, blood pressure is taken toward the end of each exercise level.

FUNCTIONAL CLASS	CLINICAL STATUS	O₂ REQUIREMENTS ml O₂/kg/min	STEP TEST NAGLE, BALKE, NAUGHTON 2 min stages 30 steps/min	BRUCE 3-min stages mph %gr	KATTUS 3-min stages mph %gr	BALKE % grade at 3.4 mph	BALKE % grade at 3 mph	BICYCLE ERGOMETER** For 70 kg body weight kgm/min
NORMAL AND I	PHYSICALLY ACTIVE SUBJECTS / SEDENTARY HEALTHY	56.0	(Step height increased 4 cm q 2 min)			26		
		52.5				24		
		49.0			4 22	22		1500
		45.5	Height (cm)	4.2 16		20		
		42.0	40		4 18	18	22.5	1350
		38.5	36			16	20.0	1200
		35.0	32		4 14	14	17.5	1050
		31.5	28	3.4 14		12	15.0	900
		28.0	24		4 10	10	12.5	750
II	DISEASED, RECOVERED / SYMPTOMATIC PATIENTS	24.5	20	2.5 12	3 10	8	10.0	
		21.0	16			6	7.5	600
		17.5	12	1.7 10	2 10	4	5.0	450
III		14.0	8			2	2.5	300
		10.5	4				0.0	
		7.0						150
IV		3.5						

Figure 3-3. Functional class, clinical status, and corresponding oxygen requirements for various exercise tests in clinical use (reproduced by permission from The Committee on Exercise: "Exercise Testing and Training of Apparently Healthy Individuals: A Handbook for Physicians," American Heart Association, Dallas, 1972, p. 13.)

Table 3-1.   Age-Predicted Maximal and Submaximal Heart
             Rates

Age	Maximal H. R.	75% Max. H. R.	85% Max. H. R.	90% Max. H. R.
20	197	148	167	177
25	195	146	166	175
30	193	145	164	173
35	191	143	162	172
40	189	142	161	170
45	187	140	159	168
50	184	138	156	166
55	182	136	155	164
60	180	135	153	162
65	178	133	151	160
70	176	132	150	158
75	174	130	148	157
80	172	129	146	155
85	170	127	145	153

MASTER'S TWO-STEP TEST

This test has gradually been replaced by the graded exercise
test using either a treadmill or bicycle. This is still useful as
a screening test, however, if one is not equipped to do more
sophisticated exercise tests. A standard set of steps are used,
and the patient walks up and down the steps during a 3-minute
period, the number of trips being determined by a chart based
on age and weight. Electrocardiographic and blood pressure
monitoring is not performed during the test, but the electrocardiogram (utilizing leads II, V_4, V_5, and V_6) is recorded
immediately and at 2 and 6 minutes after completion of the test.

COMPARATIVE PHYSIOLOGY OF EXERCISE TESTS

A comparison of the oxygen requirements, relative functional
class and clinical status for completion of progressive stages of
various exercise tests is shown in Figure 3-3.

Table 3-2.   Bruce Multistage Exercise Test

Stage	Minutes	Speed (MPH)	Grade (%)
1	3	1.7	10
2	3	2.5	12
3	3	3.4	14
4	3	4.2	16
5	3	5.0	18
6	3	5.5	20
7	3	6.0	22

INDICATIONS FOR DISCONTINUATION OF THE STRESS TEST

1. Achievement of maximum (or submaximum) predicted heart rate
2. Fatigue
3. Faintness, dizziness, ataxia, or severe dyspnea
4. Severe chest pain
5. Development of significant ventricular ectopy (frequent PVCs, PVC couplets, or runs of ventricular tachycardia)
6. Development of heart block
7. Development of hypotension or significant drop in blood pressure
8. Severe leg claudication
9. Development of clamminess and cold skin
10. Severe hypertension
11. Development of marked ST segment changes

INTERPRETATION OF THE STRESS TEST

The following parameters are assessed following completion of the exercise test (treadmill, bicycle, or step):

1. Duration of exercise
2. Heart rate response
3. Blood pressure response
4. Clinical response
5. Development of arrhythmias
6. ST segment changes
7. R, T, and U wave changes

CLINICAL RESPONSE TO EXERCISE

The duration of exercise as well as the heart rate and blood pressure responses are indicators of the physical condition of the patient as well as the presence or absence of cardiovascular disease. Those individuals in better physical condition will be able to exercise longer at a lower heart rate and blood pressure for the same level of exercise as individuals who are deconditioned or in poor condition. Failure to increase systolic blood pressure or heart rate appropriately, or even more important, a fall in systolic blood pressure with progressive exercise is usually an indication of significant cardiovascular compromise and may indicate left main or triple-vessel coronary artery disease.

If symptoms occur during or following the exercise test, the time of development of symptoms should be noted for later correlation with the electrocardiogram. It should also be noted whether the symptoms improve or worsen with further exercise and how long it takes for the symptoms to subside after exercise is terminated.

The patient should be examined prior to and following exercise for evidence of abnormalities of heart sounds, presence of murmurs, presence of S4 or S3 gallop, presence of systolic clicks, and the presence of bruits over the major arteries. The development of an S4 or S3 gallop or a decrease in intensity of the first heart sound following exercise are all indicators of the development of left ventricular dysfunction and suggests the presence of significant coronary artery disease.

ARRHYTHMIAS DURING EXERCISE

If arrhythmias occur, it should also be noted whether the arrhythmia improves or worsens with further exercise as well as what changes occur in the arrhythmia following termination of exercise. PVCs which occur at rest and decrease with exercise or PVCs which occur only at a very high heart rate tend to be benign in nature. PVCs associated with coronary artery disease or other cardiac pathology tend to occur with mild to moderate exercise and tend to increase in frequency and severity with further exercise.

INTERPRETATION OF THE
STRESS ELECTROCARDIOGRAM

ST Segment Changes

The key to the identification of ischemia from the exercise
stress test is the ST segment of the electrocardiogram. Normally, the ST segment is isoelectric to the QRS segment, while
an ischemic type of ST segment is usually defined as a down-
ward displacement of at least 0.1 mv (equal to 1 mm displacement with standard calibration of 1 mv = 10 mm) of either
horizontal or negative slope and of at least .06 sec duration
(Figure 3-4B, C). Although upsloping ST segment depression
("J point" depression) had in the past been felt to be a normal
or nondiagnostic type of response to exercise (Figure 3-4D),
most cardiologists now feel that a slowly upsloping segment
(Figure 3-4E) is also an abnormal response. In order to distinguish an abnormal from a normal upsloping ST segment, it
is necessary to measure either the slope of the ST segment or,
more easily, the amount of ST segment depression at 0.08 sec
after the J point (the J point is defined as the junction between
the end of the QRS and the beginning of the ST segment). Depression of at least 1.5 mm at this point would be considered
an abnormal response.
    ST segment changes can occur during exercise and normalize
during the recovery period or sometimes occur only after termination of exercise and when the patient is supine. In some cases
the degree of ST segment depression can even increase during
the recovery period. Any of these types of responses is considered abnormal; however, a borderline abnormal response
which occurs at peak exercise and quickly normalizes with recovery is probably of less significance than the other types of
responses. Using ST segment depression alone as the criterion
for positivity of the test results in an average sensitivity of
detection of coronary artery disease of approximately 70% in a
middle-aged population.
    ST segment elevation with exercise (Figure 3-4G) is another
type of abnormal response which is seen much less commonly
than ST segment depression but is of important diagnostic value
when it does occur. Such a finding often indicates the presence
of either critical coronary artery disease or (in the presence of
diagnostic Q waves) the presence of a left ventricular aneurysm.
    False-positive ST segment depression (defined as a positive
stress test in the absence of the demonstrable coronary artery
disease) can be due to multiple causes, including resting ECG
abnormalities, left bundle or right bundle branch block,

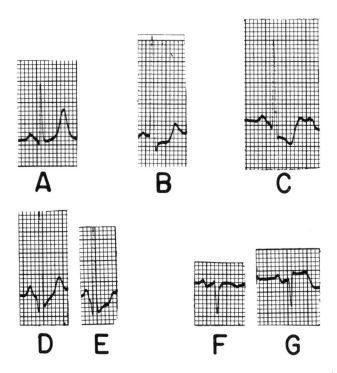

Figure 3-4.   Examples of ECG responses to stress testing.
(A) Normal, isoelectric ST segment; (B) significant horizontal
ST depression; (C) significant downsloping ST depression;
(D) nonsignificant upsloping "J" point depression; (E) possibly
significant upsloping "J" point depression (at 0. 08 seconds after
the "J" point, there is 1. 5 mm depression; (F) V_1 lead before;
and (G) after exercise, illustrating abnormal ST elevation with
exercise.

left ventricular hypertrophy, digitalis, hypokalemia, mitral
valve prolapse syndrome, and Wolff-Parkinson-White (WPW)
syndrome. If there is baseline (preexercise) ST segment depression, or ST segment depression develops with hyperventilation or with Valsalva maneuver, there should be at least 1 mm
of additional ST segment depression which occurs with exercise
in order to interpret the test as positive. In general, the frequency of false-positive ST segment depression due to all causes
is about 10% in men and 30% in women.

T Wave Changes

It is not uncommon to see upright T waves become inverted with
exercise or inverted T waves to become upright. Although such
changes may accompany ischemia, they are in themselves nonspecific and should not be interpreted as ischemic in the absence
of diagnostic ST segment changes.

U Wave Changes

Although not a fequent finding, the appearance or development
of an inverted U wave after exercise is a highly specific finding
indicative of severe disease of the left anterior descending
coronary artery.

R Wave Changes

Since the height of the R wave is directly related to left ventricular volume, an increase in left ventricular volume usually results in an increase in the height of the R wave amplitude, and
a decrease in volume results in reduction of voltage. Thus it
has been recognized that in a normal individual there tends to
be no change or a reduction in left ventricular volume and R
wave voltage with exercise, while in patients with coronary
artery disease there tends to be an increase in left ventricular
volume and R wave voltage. Although an increase in R wave
voltage is a less reliable sign of coronary artery disease compared to ST segment depression, the additional information
yielded by R wave analysis may be helpful in patients with
borderline or nondiagnostic ST segment responses.

CLINICAL CHARACTERIZATION OF
CORONARY DISEASE BY STRESS TESTING

To categorize a stress test as merely positive or negative based
on the ECG response is to miss a great deal of additional useful
information contained in this test. It is now recognized that
there are degrees of positivity of the ST segment response depending upon the extent of ST segment depression, the duration
of exercise as well as the heart rate and blood pressure (double
product = peak heart rate x peak systolic pressure) at which the
positive ST segment response occurs, and the length of time
for the ST segment to return to normal after termination of
exercise. More significant coronary artery disease and a
worse prognosis is associated with early and deep ST segment
depression, particularly when it occurs at a low heart rate and/
or low blood pressure and persists well into the recovery period.

In addition to the electrocardiogram, other parameters are useful to monitor during exercise and correlate with the presence of coronary artery disease as well as with prognosis. The development of arrhythmias, S4 and S3 gallops, a mitral regurgitant murmur, or pallor and cold sweats have already been commented upon and indicate the development of left ventricular dysfunction with exercise and suggest the presence of significant coronary artery disease. The development of chest pain or other symptoms consistent with angina pectoris with exercise also gives added significance to a positive ST segment response, and a combination of significant ST segment depression and chest pain is virtually diagnostic of the presence of significant coronary artery disease.

The duration of exercise is another indicator of the presence of cardiovascular disease as well as the general fitness of the patient. It has been shown that patients who are unable to exercise for 3-4 minutes on the treadmill have a poor prognosis, whether or not ECG changes develop.

Similarly, blood pressure and heart rate response are useful indicators of cardiovascular states. Normally, systolic blood pressure should increase with exercise. A fall in blood pressure with exercise of 10 mmHg or more is often associated with severe left ventricular dysfunction during exercise and thus suggestive of severe coronary artery disease. Inability to increase systolic blood pressure to greater than 130 mmHg is also likely to be associated with left ventricular dysfunction.

Heart rate response has also been found to be a useful indicator of cardiovascular state. The inability of a patient to achieve his maximum predicted heart rate (in the absence of an interfering drug or excellent physical conditioning), termed chronotropic incompetence, has been associated with a poor prognosis.

COMBINED CRITERIA IN
INTERPRETATION OF THE STRESS TEST

The greater the number and the greater the magnitude of abnormal responses to exercise (ST segment depression or elevation, duration of exercise, blood pressure and heart rate response, symptoms and signs), the higher the likelihood of significant coronary artery disease and of greater severity of disease. In a recent study (Kansal et al.) a diagnostic scoring technique was derived based on four variables: maximal heart rate achieved and treadmill time. Using these variables, diagnostic accuracy was increased from 60% using ST depression alone to 83% in a group of men.

The prognostic as well as the diagnostic power of an exercise stress test is greatly increased by combining the electrocardiographic and clinical responses. It has been shown, for example, that patients with coronary artery disease who nonetheless have a normal ST segment response to exercise, as well as normal heart rate response and exercise duration, have a greater than 90% 4-year survival, while coronary disease patients with abnormal ST segment response, abnormal heart rate response, and abnormal exercise duration have only a 60% 4-year survival.

REFERENCES

Davidson, R. M.: Controversies in the use of exercise stress testing in the diagnosis and management of ischemic heart disease, in Corday, E. (Ed.), "Controversies in Cardiology" Cardiovascular Clinics, 8, F. A. Davis Company, Philadelphia, 1977, pp. 159-170.

Ellestad, M. H.: "Stress Testing, Principles and Practice," Ed. 2, F. A. Davis Company, Philadelphia, 1980.

Fortuin, N. J., and Weiss, J. L.: Exercise Stress Testing, in Weissler, A. M. (Ed.), "Reviews of Contemporary Laboratory Methods," American Heart Association, Inc., Dallas, 1980, pp. 157-195.

Froelicher, V. F.: Exercise testing as part of the reasonable workup before recommending medical or surgical therapy for coronary heart disease. Circulation 651 (Suppl II), 1982, II-15-20.

Froelicher, V. F.: Exercise testing and training: Clinical Applications. J Am Coll Cardiol 1, 1983, pp. 114-125.

Goldschlager, N.: Use of the treadmill test in the diagnosis of coronary artery disease in patients with chest pain. Ann Intern Med 97, 1982, pp. 383-388.

Kansal, S., Roitman, D., Bradley, E. L. Jr., and Sheffield, L. T.: Enhanced evaluation of treadmill tests by means of scoring based on multivariate analysis and its clinical application: A study of 608 points. Am J Cardiol 52, 1983, pp. 1155-1160.

McNeer, J. F., Margolis, J. R., Lee, K. L., Kisslo, J. A., Peter, R. H., Kong, Y., Behar, V. S., Wallace, A. G., McCants, C. B., and Rosati, R.: The role of the exercise test in the evaluation of patients for ischemic heart disease. Circulation 57, 1978, pp. 64-70.

Sheffield, L. T.: Exercise Stress Testing, in Braunwald, E. (Ed.), "Heart Disease," 2nd Edition, W. B. Saunders, Philadelphia, 1984, pp. 258-278.

Young, S. G., and Froelicher, V. F.: Exercise testing: An update. Mod Conc Cardiovasc Dis 52, 1983, pp. 25-28.

American College of Sports Medicine: Guidelines for Graded Exercise Testing and Exercise Prescription, 2nd Ed., Lea & Febiger, Philadelphia, 1980.

The Committee on Exercise: Exercise Testing and Training of Apparently Healthy Individuals: A Handbook for Physicians, American Heart Association, Dallas, 1972.

The Committee on Exercise: Exercise Testing and Training of Individuals with Heart Disease or at High Risk for its Development: A Handbook for Physicians, American Heart Association, Dallas, 1975.

Chapter 4

NUCLEAR STRESS TESTS

INTRODUCTION

The addition of nuclear stress testing to our diagnostic modalities has added considerably to our ability to correctly identify patients with coronary artery disease as well as to derive further information on the extent, distribution, and significance of their disease. At present, there are two major types of nuclear stress tests: (1) myocardial perfusion imaging using thallium-201 (also known as a thallium stress test) and (2) radionuclide angiography (also known as an exercise wall motion test). Although there is diagnostic overlap between these two types of tests, the selection of which test to order in a particular patient is determined by the specific clinical situation as well as by the availability of the test.

THALLIUM STRESS TEST

The principle of the thallium stress test is that intravenously injected thallium-201 is taken up only by perfused and viable myocardial cells. In a normal individual, a thallium scan shows uniform uptake throughout the myocardium. In contrast, if there are areas of either decreased perfusion due to coronary artery disease or areas of nonviable myocardium due to previous myocardial infarction, uptake of thallium will be decreased or absent in these areas.

INDICATIONS

1. In place of a standard ECG stress test in which the ECG would be uninterpretable (such as with left bundle branch block)
2. As a further diagnostic test for coronary artery disease in clinically uncertain cases such as the patient with an equivocal or uninterpretable electrocardiographic stress test

31

3. As a further diagnostic test in cases where the electro-cardiographic stress test is abnormal but other clinical indications of coronary artery disease are absent or equivocal
4. As a further diagnostic test for coronary artery disease in cases where the electrocardiographic stress test is negative but there are other strong indications of coronary artery disease
5. To determine the site and extent of stress induced ischemia
6. To differentiate areas of stress-induced ischemia from areas of prior infarction

METHOD

A standard stress test is performed, and at peak exercise level the radioisotope is injected in a peripheral vein and the patient continues to exercise for 1 more minute. At the end of this time the exercise is terminated and the patient lies down, during which time standard electrocardiographic tracings are taken and nuclear imaging is done with a gamma camera using multiple views. The imaging is repeated at 4 hours (without additional isotope injection) and, if necessary, again at 24 hours after the stress test to evaluate "redistribution" uptake of thallium.

(A recently developed alternative to exercise testing involves the use of dipyridamole [Persantine] infusion in conjunction with thallium imaging. As a powerful arteriolar dilator, this agent results in differential flow to normally perfused myocardium compared to myocardium supplied by stenotic coronary arteries. Thus, this test can be used without the need for exercise in selected patients.)

INTERPRETATION

In a normal individual, thallium uptake is uniform throughout the left ventricle, indicating normal perfusion and myocardial viability (Figure 4-1). In areas of scar (infarction), there will be absence of uptake in both the stress and redistribution images, whereas in areas of stress-induced ischemia, the stress image will show a decreased uptake immediately after stress but normal or improved uptake on the redistribution image (Figure 4-2). In addition, the "washout" rate has been found to be abnormal in ischemic areas, and this is also a useful indicator of ischemia. Furthermore, increased pulmonary uptake of thallium has been associated with significant left ventricular dysfunction (increased pulmonary venous pressure) and is still a further indication of left ventricular disease.

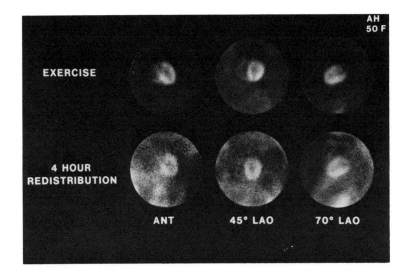

Figure 4-1. Normal thallium-201 myocardial scan. The upper
three images are the scans in the anterior, 45° LAO and 70°
LAO views immediately postexercise, while the lower three
images are the scans in the same views 4 hours after exercise
(redistribution phase). There is uniform distribution of the
isotope throughout the myocardium in the immediate and redistribution images. (Reprinted with permission from Berman,
D. S. and Mason, D. T., (Eds.), "Clinical Nuclear Cardiology,"
New York, Grune & Stratton, 1981, p. 66.)

The diagnostic sensitivity and specificity of this test is
higher than with the ordinary electrocardiographic stress test,
and it is particularly useful when the information obtained is
combined with the clinical and electrocardiographic data. A recent modification of the thallium stress test involves the use of
tomographic imaging, which provides more accurate localization
of abnormalities than does the standard imaging technique.

EXERCISE WALL MOTION TEST

In this test, blood pool imaging of the left ventricular and right
ventricular chambers is obtained using technetium-99m. Combined with exercise testing, both global and regional left ventricular and right ventricular function can be assessed at rest
and with exercise.

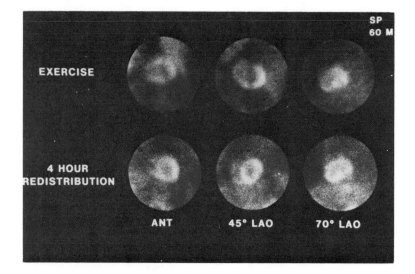

Figure 4-2.   Abnormal thallium-201 myocardial scan in a 60-
year-old man with multiple-vessel coronary artery disease
without prior myocardial infarction. There are multiple perfusion defects present in the exercise images which normalize
in the redistribution phase. In addition, the exercise images
show marked uptake of thallium in the lungs, a finding indicative of left ventricular failure during exercise. (Reprinted
with permission from Berman, D. S. and Mason, D. T. , (Eds.),
"Clinical Nuclear Cardiology," New York, Grune & Stratton,
1981, p. 67.)

INDICATIONS

1. As an alternative to the thallium test in the diagnosis of
    coronary artery disease
2. To provide additional diagnostic information in conjunc-
    tion with the thallium test
3. When it is desirable to determine ventricular function at
    rest and with exercise

METHODS

As in the thallium test, this test is usually (but not necessarily)
combined with an exercise stress test. Because imaging must
be done during exercise as well as afterwards, the test is usually
done with a bicycle rather than a treadmill to minimize motion
of the upper torso. If more than one view is desired, a separate

exercise test is done for each view. In patients unable to exercise, the test may be done in conjunction with atrial pacing to increase the heart rate. Either of two imaging techniques can be utilized and both are in common use: (1) In the "first pass" technique, the isotope is imaged as a bolus injection of technetium-99m passes through the heart. Separate injections of the isotope are given prior to exercise and during exercise for this purpose. (2) In the other technique, known as equilibrium or ECG-gated ("multiple-gated acquisition" or MUGA), only one injection is necessary, and multiple images are timed (gated) to correspond with the ECG and summated by computer techniques to produce multiple systolic and diastolic images. In each technique, images are provided which are analogous to a contrast left ventriculogram in which the contraction pattern of both the right and left ventricles can be visualized and automated analysis of global ventricular function (ejection fraction) and regional wall motion can be easily derived. Imaging can be done in each stage of exercise, but in only one view per study.

INTERPRETATION

In a normal individual both the left ventricle and right ventricle contract uniformly at rest and with exercise, with an increase in ejection fraction occurring with exercise (Figure 4-3). A variety of patterns can be seen in heart disease. In very mild ischemic heart disease a normal pattern may also be seen, but with increasing severity of ischemic heart disease, the left ventricular ejection fraction fails to increase with exercise, and with severe disease the ejection fraction almost always decreases with exercise compared to rest. (This pattern, however, is not specific for ischemic heart disease and may occur in other forms of heart disease.) In patients with coronary artery disease but without prior infarction, the left ventricular contraction pattern is generally normal at rest but becomes abnormal with exercise in areas of the left ventricle supplied by stenotic coronary vessels (Figure 4-4). In areas of prior infarction (scar), wall motion is generally abnormal both at rest and with exercise. In nonischemic forms of heart disease wall motion abnormalities (when present) tend to involve the entire left ventricle in a uniform manner, whereas in ischemic heart disease the wall motion abnormalities tend to be segmental, involving only portions of the left ventricle supplied by stenotic or occluded coronary arteries. As in thallium testing, it is usually possible to determine both the location and extent of significant coronary artery disease with this technique.

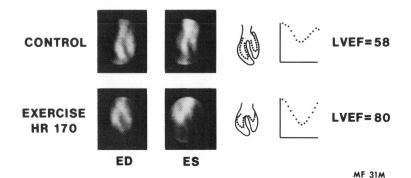

Figure 4-3. Normal exercise wall motion study (MUGA scan) showing end-diastolic (ED) and end-systolic (ES) frames in the left ventricular oblique (LAO) view (left); superimposed traced end-diastolic and end-systolic right ventricular and left ventricular outlines (middle); and time-count curves (right) during the control (resting) and exercise states. A normal response is seen, with uniform contraction patterns for both ventricles at rest with increased contraction during exercise (left ventricular ejection fraction LVEF increases from 58% to 80%). (Reprinted with permission from Berman, D. S. and Mason, D. T., (Eds.), "Clinical Nuclear Cardiology," New York, Grune & Stratton, 1981, p. 251.)

ADVANTAGES AND LIMITATIONS
OF NUCLEAR STRESS TESTING

As indicated, both the thallium stress test and the exercise wall motion test provide information beyond that which is provided by the exercise electrocardiographic stress test in regard to the presence, location, and extent of coronary artery disease. Both tests can be done as outpatient procedures, and the images are computer processed, providing objective measurements. The diagnostic accuracy in detection of coronary disease is similar for both tests. It should be noted however, that there are several disadvantages to these tests. Although their accuracy in diagnosing ischemic heart disease is greater than electrocardiographic stress testing, these tests are still not 100% accurate, and they can result in both false-positive and false-negative tests for a variety of reasons. Moreover, both tests are expensive and require considerable equipment and personnel to perform and interpret, and they do expose the patient to a small amount of radiation. Furthermore, both tests require the cooperation of the patient and the ability of the patient to perform

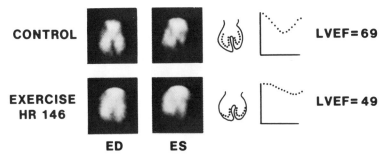

CONTROL   LVEF= 69

EXERCISE HR 146   LVEF= 49

ED   **ES**

HK 71M

Figure 4-4. Abnormal exercise wall motion study in a patient with triple-vessel coronary artery disease without prior myocardial infarction (the format is the same as in Figure 4-3). Wall motion is normal at rest, with a normal LVEF of 69%, but is abnormal during exercise, with a fall in LVEF to 49%. (Reprinted with permission from Berman, D. S. and Mason, D. T. , (Eds.), "Clinical Nuclear Cardiology," New York, Grune & Stratton, 1981, p. 252.)

strenous exercise in order to achieve meaningful results, although the recently developed dipyridamole thallium test may obviate the need for exercise.

REFERENCES

Beller, G. A.: Radionuclide techniques in the evaluation of the patient with chest pain. Mod Conc Cardiovasc Dis 50, 1981, pp. 43-48.

Berger, B. C. , and Brest, A. N.: Exercise electrocardiography and stress thallium-201 imaging in coronary artery disease, in Fowler, N. D. (Ed.), "Noninvasive Diagnostic Methods in Cardiology," Cardiovascular Clinics, Brest, A. N. (Ed.), F. A. Davis Company, Philadelphia, 1983, pp. 253-277.

Berger, H. J. , and Zaret, B. L.: Nuclear cardiology. N Engl J Med 305, 1981, pp. 799-807, pp. 855-865.

Berman, D. S. , and Mason, D. T. (Eds.): "Clinical Nuclear Cardiology," Grune & Stratton, New York, 1981.

Bodenheimer, M. M. , and Helfant, R. H. : Exercise radio-nuclide angiography: role in diagnosis and management of cardiovascular disease, in Fowler, N. O. (Ed.), "Noninvasive Diagnostic Methods in Cardiology," Cardiovascular Clinics, Brest, A. N. (Ed.), F. A. Davis Company, Philadelphia, 1983, pp. 243-252.

Corbett, J. R. , Redish, G. , Gabliani, G. , Jansen, D. , Filip-chuk, N. , Lewis, S. E. , and Willerson, J. T. : Noninvasive myocardial scintigraphic assessment of the patient with chest pain. Cardiovasc Rev Rep 5, 1984, pp. 119-137.

Elkayam, U. , Weinstein, M. , Berman, D. , Maddahi, J. , Staniloff, H. , Freeman, M. , Waxman, A. , Swan, H. J. C. , and Forrester, J. : Stress thallium-201 myocardial scintigraphy and exercise technetium ventriculography in the detection and location of chronic coronary artery disease: comparison of sensitivity and specificity of these noninvasive tests alone and in combination. Am Heart J 101, 1981, pp. 657-666.

Ellestad, M. H. : "Stress Testing, Principles and Practice," 2nd Ed. , F. A. Davis Company, Philadelphia, 1980, pp. 291-301.

Gibson, R. S. , and Watson, D. D. : Clinical applications of myocardial perfusion scintigraphy with thallium-201, in Yu, P. N. , and Goodwin, T. F. (Eds.), "Progress in Cardiology," 12, Lea and Febiger, Philadelphia, 1983, pp. 67-112.

Osbakken, M. D. , Okada, R. D. , Boucher, C. A. , Strauss, H. W. , and Pohost, G. M. : Comparison of exercise perfusion and ventricular function imaging: An analysis of factors affecting the diagnostic accuracy of each technique. J Am Coll Cardiol 3, 1984, pp. 272-283.

Pitt, B. , and Thrall, J. H. : Evaluation of patients with ischemic heart disease by thallium-201 myocardial imaging. Am Heart J 103, 1982.

Pitt, B. , Kalff, V. , Rabinovitch, M. A. , Buda, A. J. , Colfer, H. T. , Vogel, R. A. , and Thrall, J. H. : Impact of radio-nuclide techniques on evaluation of patients with ischemic heart disease. J Am Coll Cardiol 1, 1983, pp. 63-72.

Wagner, H. N. : Nuclear techniques in ischemic heart disease. Am Heart J 103, 1982, pp. 681-688.

Zaret, B. L. , and Berger, H. J. : Radionuclide studies of ventricular performance in coronary artery disease, in Yu, P. N. , and Goodwin, T. F. (Eds.), "Progress in Cardiology," 12, Lea and Febiger, Philadelphia, 1983, pp. 33-66.

Chapter 5

OTHER NONINVASIVE TESTS IN THE DIAGNOSIS
OF CORONARY ARTERY DISEASE

CARDIAC FLUOROSCOPY

Fluoroscopy of the heart, using an image intensification system, is a highly useful technique for the detection of coronary artery disease, particularly in clinically questionable cases. The demonstration of calcification within one or more coronary arteries is a very good indication of the presence of significant coronary artery disease, particularly in younger patients. In older patients (70 years or older) the test is less specific than in patients 50 years or younger. Unfortunately, flouroscopy for coronary calcification is not a very sensitive test, and failure to find demonstrable calcification certainly does not rule out the presence of significant coronary artery disease.

ECHOCARDIOGRAPHY

Although echocardiography has not generally been utilized to a great extent in the assessment of coronary artery disease, it does have a role in the evaluation of patients with ischemic heart disease, particularly when the two-dimensional technique is used. With this technique, the left ventricle (as well as the other chambers) can be visualized, and left ventricular contraction pattern and wall thickening can be easily assessed to identify areas of segmental dysfunction consistent with previous myocardial infarction or severe ischemia. Left ventricular aneurysms and intracavitary mural thrombi can be easily detected. The demonstration of resting segmental wall motion abnormality can be a very helpful sign in a patient with suspected ischemic heart disease, particularly when the electrocardiogram is nondiagnostic or normal. Moreover, echocardiography does not involve radiation and can be performed on patients (either in an outpatient or inpatient setting) in a matter of 15 to 20 minutes. In addition, with a good quality two-dimensional echocardiogram, it is often possible to visualize the origins of the left main and sometimes the right coronary artery. Unfortunately, however, the sensitivity and specificity of this technique in detecting lesions within the coronary arteries are too low with present techniques to be a generally useful clinical tool for the detection of coronary disease.

CARDIOKYMOGRAPHY (CKG)

Cardiokymography is a relatively new technique that is becoming increasingly available in the diagnosis of coronary artery disease. This technique detects cardiac wall motion by changes in an electromagnetic field generated by a small transducer placed on the chest wall. By distinguishing between normal (inward) and abnormal (outward) systolic motion, left ventricular wall motion abnormalities can often be detected. When combined with an exercise test, the sensitivity and specificity of this technique are said to approach that of thallium stress testing. Clinical experience with this technique have been limited thus far, and more extensive testing will need to be done to make this a standard diagnostic tool.

HOLTER MONITORING

Twenty-four hour continuous ambulatory ECG (Holter) monitoring can be a highly useful test in the diagnosis of ischemic heart disease. As in the ECG stress test, both symptomatic and asymptomatic ischemia can be detected by analysis of the ST segments. Whereas the stress test provokes ischemia by (unnatural) brief and intense exercise, the Holter device monitors the electrocardiographic response to normal activity and stress. It is particularly useful in detecting episodes of rest angina, including variant (Prinzmetal's) angina. In order to maximize the diagnostic accuracy of this technique, a two-channel system with good frequency response should be utilized. It should be recognized, however, that false-positive ST segment changes are relatively common with this technique, so that the diagnostic accuracy of detecting ischemia is less than with ECG stress testing. The development of ST segment changes on an ambulatory ECG recorder therefore generally need to be confirmed as significant by at least one other diagnostic test.

NEW DIAGNOSTIC IMAGING METHODS:
CT, NMR, PET, AND DSA

In the past few years, a whole new variety of imaging techniques has been developed which are being applied to cardiac diagnosis. These include computerized tomography (CT), nuclear magnetic resonance (NMR), positron emission tomography (PET), and digital subtraction angiography (DSA). The current role for each of these techniques in routine cardiac evaluations is still very limited, with the future potential being very promising but, as yet, uncertain. Each technique and its current applications will therefore be discussed only briefly.

CT

Computerized tomography has been utilized for brain imaging since 1972, and for imaging of the abdomen and other parts of the body more recently. Because of the speed limitation of CT scanners until very recently, however, a contracting heart could not be imaged very well. With the new generation of equipment and the use of ECG gating, however, this limitation has been overcome, and cardiac imaging is now readily accomplishable. In conjunction with intravenously administered contrast material, CT provides detailed reconstructed three-dimensional images of cardiac anatomy including chamber sizes and shape and is particularly suited for imaging left ventricular aneurysms and intracavitary clots. It can also differentiate infarcted from normal myocardium and can image coronary bypass grafts and evaluate graft patency (although graft stenosis cannot be determined). Moreover, this technique can be used for determining ejection fraction and regional wall motion. At the present time, several new types of CT scanners are being developed specifically for cardiac imaging, and may eventually allow visualization of the coronary arteries. As of now, CT imaging of the heart is feasible and may even be practical, and complements other noninvasive techniques more than it offers new capabilities.

NMR

This technique is still largely in the investigative state but has been shown to provide detailed images of cardiac anatomy similar to CT scans. As with CT, chamber size and shape are well visualized, and areas of myocardial infarction, ventricular aneurysms, and mural thrombi can be identified. In addition, areas of abnormal flow pattern, resultant from abnormal wall motion, can also be seen. Proximal portions of coronary arteries have also been visualized. In common with CT scanner, NMR equipment is very expensive (1 million to over 2 million dollars). Unlike CT scanning (and nuclear scanning), NMR does not involve radiation exposure or injection of contrast agents. In addition to cost of acquisition, however, there are several other disadvantages that will limit the routine clinical application of this technique for most facilities: The site preparation, staff, and maintenance are very expensive, and the equipment cannot be used in proximity to any metallic objects, including implanted pacemakers and other metallic implants.

PET

Although a discussion of the physics involved is beyond the scope of this text, PET imaging differs in a number of ways from standard nuclear imaging. By using positron emitting radioisotopes (such as oxygen-15, N-13 ammonia, C-11 palmitate, rubidium-82, and others), in conjunction with a positron tomography camera, information about cardiac function not obtainable with other techniques can be derived, including myocardial oxygen utilization and myocardial metabolism, in addition to myocardial ischemia. As with other techniques, ventricular size and function can also be determined as well as myocardial perfusion. A different isotope is necessary for each type of study. Unfortunately, most of the isotopes need to be prepared with an on-site cyclotron, thus limiting the practicality of this technique. Perhaps even more than the other techniques described in this section, PET imaging is likely to remain primarily a research tool for the near future.

DSA

Although also a very new development, digital subtraction angiography is already being applied clinically to the evaluation of ischemic heart disease (as well as to other forms of cardiovascular disease). It is a semiinvasive technique in that it involves the injection of radiographic contrast material. Because contrast can be given intravenously or in small amounts by direct intraarterial injection, it can be used in virtually any application that makes use of standard angiography without the need for selective arterial cannulation. Thus left ventriculograms and aortograms are easily obtainable and may become bedside procedures with the availability of portable equipment. Assessment of bypass graft patency can be done with a nonselective aortic root injection (Figure 5-1). Although

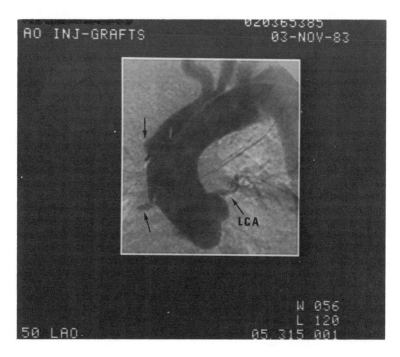

Figure 5-1. Aortic root angiogram obtained by DSA, illustrating
two obstructed saphenous vein coronary bypass grafts (arrows)
and the initial portion of the left coronary artery (LCA).

nonselective coronary arteriograms are still not of comparable
diagnostic quality to selective angiography, this is a potentially
very important development for this technique. At the present
time, high resolution selective coronary arteriograms are obtainable by direct injection of contrast into a coronary artery
ostium (Figure 5-2). In conjunction with computer analysis
techniques, coronary lesions can be measured more precisely
than is possible with routine visual analysis of cineangiograms.
In addition, computer techniques used in conjunction with DSA
coronary arteriography can provide additional information on
coronary flow which may be clinically useful.

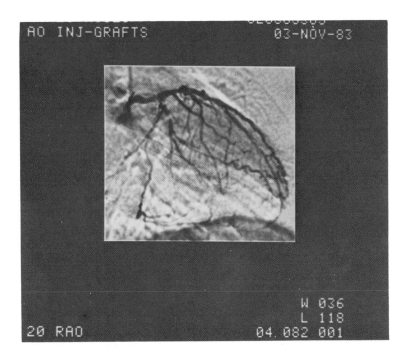

Figure 5-2. Selective left coronary arteriogram obtained by DSA in a patient with multiple coronary lesions.

REFERENCES

FLUOROSCOPY

Aldrich, R. G. , Brensike, J. F. , Battaghini, J. W. , Richardson, J. M. , Loh, I. K. , Stone, N. J. , Passamani, E. R. , Ackerstein, H. , Seningen, R. , Borer, J. S. , Levy, R. I. , and Epstein, S. E. : Coronary calcifications in the detection of coronary artery disease and comparison with electrocardiographic exercise testing. Circulation, 59, 1979, pp. 1113-1114.

Bartel, A. G. , Chen, J. T. T. , Peter, R. H. , Behar, V. S. , Kong, Y. , and Lester, R. G. : The significance of coronary calcification detected by fluoroscopy. A report of 360 patients. Circulation 49, 1970, pp. 1247-1253.

ECHOCARDIOGRAPHY

Charuzi, Y. , Davidson, R. M. , Barrett, M. J. , Beeder, C. ,
Marshall, L. A. , Loh, I. K. , Prause, J. , Meerbaum, S. , and
Corday, E. : Simultaneous assessment of segmental and global
left ventricular function by two-dimensional echocardiography
in acute myocardial infarction. Clin Cardiol 6, 1983, pp. 255-
264.

Davidson, R. M. : Ischemic heart disease and left ventricular
function, in Schapira, J. N. , Charuzi, Y. , and Davidson,
R. M. (Eds.): "Two Dimension Echocardiography," Williams
& Wilkins, Baltimore, 1982, pp. 175-195.

Wann, L. S. , Faris, J. V. , Childress, R. H. , Dillon, J. C. ,
Weyman, A. E. , and Feigenbaum, H. : Exercise cross-
sectional echocardiography in ischemic heart disease. Circulation 60, 1979, pp. 1300-1308.

CARDIOKYMOGRAPHY

Silverberg, R. A. , Diamond, G. A. , Vas, R. , Tzivoni, D. ,
Swan, H. J. C. , and Forrester, J. S. : Noninvasive diagnosis
of coronary artery disease: The cardiokymographic stress test.
Circulation 61, 1980, pp. 579-589.

Weiner, D. A. , McCabe, C. H. , Dagostino, G. , Cutler, S. S. ,
and Ryan, T. J. : Cardiokymography during exercise testing:
A new device for the detection of coronary artery disease and
left ventricular wall motion abnormalities. Am J Cardiol 1983,
pp. 1307-1311.

HOLTER MONITORING

Armstrong, W. F. and Morris, S. N. : The ST segment during
ambulatory electrocardiographic monitoring. Ann Intern Med 98,
1983, pp. 249-250.

Tzivoni, D. , Stern, Z. , and Stern, S. : Transient ischemic
changes in patients with coronary artery disease while awake
and asleep, in Corday, E. and Swan, H. J. C. (Eds.), "Clinical
Strategies in Ischemic Heart Disease," Williams & Wilkins,
Baltimore, 1979, pp. 190-197.

COMPUTERIZED TOMOGRAPHY

Lipton, M. J. , Brundage, B. H. , Higgins, C. B. , and Boyd, D. P. : CT Scanning of the Heart, in Fowler, N. O. (Ed.), "Noninvasive Diagnostic Methods in Cardiology," Cardiovascular Clinics, 13/3, 1983, F. A. Davis Company, Philadelphia, pp. 385-401.

Wittenberg, J. : Computed tomography of the body (second of two parts). N Engl J Med 309, 1983, pp. 1224-1229.

NUCLEAR MAGNETIC RESONANCE

Higgins, C. B. , Lanzer, P. , Stark, D. , Botvinick, E. , Schiller, N. B. , Crooks, L. , Kaufman, L. , and Lipton, M. J.: Imaging by nuclear magnetic resonance in patients with chronic ischemic heart disease. Circulation 69, 1984, pp. 523-531.

Pohost, G. M. : Nuclear magnetic resonance. Potential applications in clinical cardiology. JAMA 251, 1984, pp. 1304-1309.

Ratner, A. V. , Pohost, G. M. , Goldman, M. R. , and Okada, R. D. : Proton Nuclear Magnetic Resonance Imaging of the Heart, in Yu, P. N. and Goodwin, J. F. (Eds.), "Progress in Cardiology," 12, Lea & Febiger, Philadelphia, 1983, pp. 135-146.

POSITRON EMISSION TOMOGRAPHY

Goldstein, R. A. , Mullani, M. A. , and Gould, K. L.: Quantitative myocardial imaging with positron emitters, in Yu, P. N. and Goodwin, J. F. (Eds.), "Progress in Cardiology," 12, Lea & Febiger, Philadelphia, 1983, pp. 147-191.

Mullani, N. A. and Gould, K. L. : Functional cardiac imaging: Positron emission tomography. Hosp Pract 19, 1984, pp. 103-118.

DIGITAL SUBTRACTION ANGIOGRAPHY

Higgins, C. B. , Mancini, G. B. J. , Norris, S. L. , and Slutsky, R. A.: Digital subtraction angiography: Technique and cardiac applications, in Yu, P. N. and Goodwin, J. F. (Eds.), "Progress in Cardiology," 12, Lea & Febiger, Philadelphia, 1983, pp. 113-133.

Myerowitz, P. D. : Digital subtraction angiography: Present and future uses in cardiovascular diagnosis. Clin Cardiol 5, 1982, pp. 623-629.

Chapter 6

CARDIAC CATHETERIZATION AND CORONARY ARTERIOGRAPHY

Coronary arteriography still remains the definitive test for the diagnosis and characterization of coronary artery disease. Although the test is invasive and carries a small but definite risk, the information derived from it far outweighs the risk in appropriately selected cases.

LEFT AND RIGHT HEART CATHETERIZATION

Catheterization of the left ventricle is usually done in conjunction with coronary arteriography for the purpose of measuring left ventricular end-diastolic pressure and for left ventricular contrast angiography. The latter, done either as a single plane right anterior oblique (RAO) view or in biplane views (RAO and left anterior oblique), demonstrate left ventricular size and shape (and allow calculation of volume and ejection fraction) as well as left ventricular contraction pattern and assessment for mitral regurgitation.

Right heart catheterization is sometimes done in conjunction with left heart catheterization and coronary arteriography, when it is desirable to measure right heart pressures, oxygen saturations, and cardiac output. This is generally done when there is an indication of heart failure or valvular disease or an intracardiac shunt is suspected.

CORONARY ARTERIOGRAPHY

INDICATIONS

The usual indications for performing coronary arteriography in patients with suspected or known coronary artery disease are as follows:

1. Patients in whom the diagnosis of coronary artery disease is still in question after noninvasive testing
2. Patients in whom the definitive diagnosis is essential

3. Patients in whom coronary artery spasm is suspected
4. Patients in whom the diagnosis is clear, but it is important to determine the extent and degree of disease
5. Patients being considered for coronary artery bypass surgery, coronary angioplasty, or other cardiac surgery

METHODS

Two techniques of coronary arteriography are currently in use and differ mainly in the approach to the peripheral artery. The risk as well as the information derived are comparable for both techniques and the choice is primarily determined by the preference and experience of the arteriographer and by the patency of the femoral and aortoiliac arteries. In the Sones technique, an incision is made in the right antecubital fossa, and the right brachial artery is opened by an incision and a specifically designed catheter is inserted into the artery and directed under fluoroscopy into the ostia of the left and right coronary arteries. At the conclusion of the procedure, the arteriotomy and skin incisions are repaired by suturing, and the patient is free to ambulate afterward. A recent modification of this technique utilizes a percutaneous approach to the brachial artery, thus avoiding the need for an arteriotomy and repair. In the alternative Judkins approach, preshaped left and right coronary artery catheters are inserted into the femoral artery in the groin by means of a percutaneous approach and no incisions or repairs are necessary, but the puncture site in the artery seals by application of firm pressure over the site, and the patient is required to keep his leg immobile for 5 to 6 hours afterward and is usually kept in bed until the next day. In each technique, multiple views of each artery are filmed using cineangiographic cameras while radiographic contrast material is injected.

INTERPRETATION

Interpretation of coronary arteriograms requires a level of expertise in this subspecialty of cardiology as well as the availability of high quality angiograms. Although there can be a great deal of normal variation in anatomy, normally there are separate left and right coronary arteries, with the left coronary being the larger system, having two main branches from the left main coronary artery—the left anterior descending artery, which supplies the anterolateral walls and apex of the left ventricle as well as most of the interventricular septum; and the circumflex branch, which supplies the posterior and posterolateral walls (Figure 6-1A). Each of these vessels has

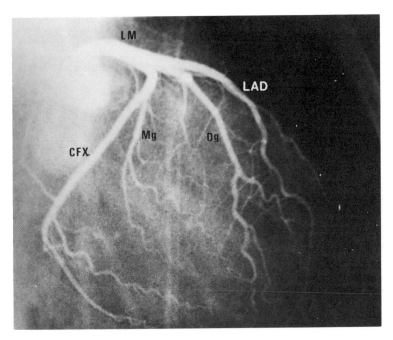

Figure 6-1A. Normal coronary arteriogram.   (A) Left coronary artery, RAO view.   LM = left main coronary artery, LAD = left anterior descending coronary artery, Dg = diagonal branch of LAD, CFX = circumflex coronary artery, Mg = marginal branch of CFX.   (B) Right coronary artery.

additional branches such as the septal and diagonal branches of the left anterior descending artery and the marginal branches of the circumflex artery.   In about 20% of cases the circumflex coronary artery supplies the posterior descending artery to the inferior wall of the left ventricle, while in the other 80% this vessel is a branch of the right coronary artery.   The right coronary artery (Figure 6-1B) supplies the inferior and part of the posterior wall of the left ventricle as well as the right ventricle.

The terminology of "single," "double," and "triple" coronary artery disease refers to the presence of disease in one, two, or all three main branches: the left anterior descending, circumflex, and right coronary artery.   The term "left main disease" refers to disease in the left main coronary artery. Disease can be confined to a single portion of a vessel or to multiple portions of one or more vessels, or can diffusely involve any or all of the arteries (Figures 6-2, 6-3).   The

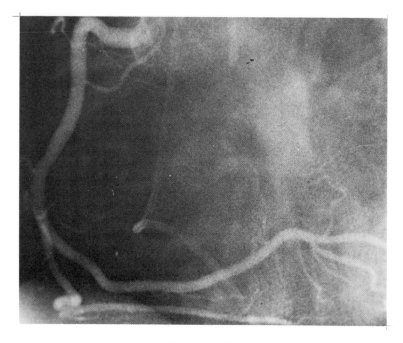

Figure 6-1B.

severity of any given lesion can be defined by estimating the percentage of narrowing of the intraluminal diameter of the vessel, or it can be described in more general terms as "mild," "moderate," or "severe" disease. In general, a lesion of less than 50% narrowing is termed mild and not felt to be functionally significant, while a lesion of 50-70% is termed moderate and is thought to be functionally significant, and a lesion of greater than 70% is felt to be severe. The prognosis if any given patient with coronary artery disease relates directly to the extent and severity of coronary artery disease demonstrable by coronary arteriography as well as to the extent of left ventricular dysfunction, demonstrable by left ventriculography. The coronary arteriogram is mandatory for all patients being considered by coronary bypass surgery, to assess not only the appropriateness for surgery, but also to decide which vessels to bypass.

When coronary artery spasm is clinically suspected and the coronary arteriogram reveals normal anatomy, a provocative test is usually done in conjunction with the arteriographic procedure: during continuous monitoring of clinical state, electrocardiogram, and arterial pressure, small incremental amounts

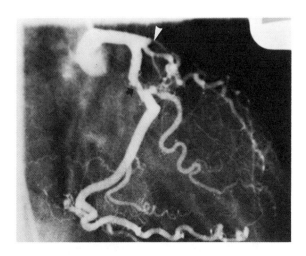

Figure 6-2. Abnormal left coronary arteriogram (RAO view) showing total occlusion of proximal LAD (white arrow) and partial occlusion of proximal CFX (black arrow).

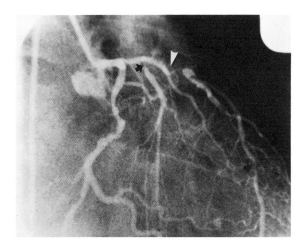

Figure 6-3. Abnormal left coronary arteriogram (RAO view) showing multiple lesions in the CFX and LAD arteries including near total obstruction at the origin of a large septal branch (left arrow) and in the proximal LAD (middle arrow). A high-grade lesion also exists in a more distal portion of the LAD (right arrow).

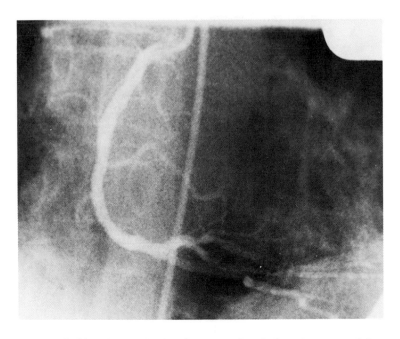

Figure 6-4A.   An example of ergonovine-induced spasm of the
right coronary artery in a patient with spontaneous episodes of
Prinzmetal's angina.   (A) LAO view of the RCA prior to ergonovine; (B) Total occlusion of the RCA in its midportion following
the intravenous administration of a total of 0.375 mg ergonovine
(in divided doses); (C) Following the intracoronary administration of 100 μg nitroglycerine the spasm is relieved and the
artery is reopened.

of ergonovine maleate are injected intravenously in an attempt
to artificially stimulate coronary spasm.   A positive test, felt
to be confirmatory of spontaneous spasm, consists of reproduc-
tion of the patient's usual chest pain in conjunction with ST segment elevation on the ECG and transient localized severe
narrowing of a coronary artery (Figure 6-4).   An intracoronary
injection of nitroglycerin is sometimes necessary to reverse
the spasm.   A negative test reveals no clinical or electrocardiographic evidence of ischemia and either no narrowing of any of
the coronary arteries or mild diffuse narrowing.   (The development of chest pain without ECG changes or demonstrable spasm
of a coronary artery may indicate esophageal spasm induced by
ergonovine.)

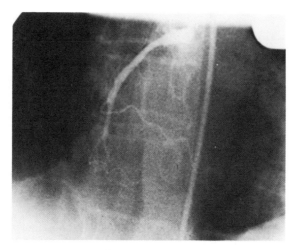

Figure 6-4B.

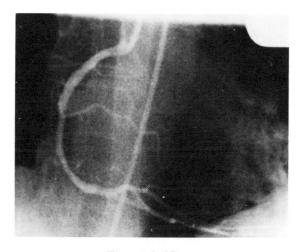

Figure 6-4C.

COMPLICATIONS AND LIMITATIONS
OF CORONARY ARTERIOGRAPHY

The obvious disadvantage of coronary arteriography is the invasive nature and need for hospitalization (although outpatient catheterizations are now also being done). The procedure is done under local anesthesia and is usually only minimally uncomfortable. The overall mortality rate of coronary arteriography is 0.1%, and the risk of myocardial infarction during the procedure is about 0.2%. Other potentially serious but uncommon complications include cerebrovascular accidents or other embolic events, and coronary artery dissection. More common but less serious complications include hematoma or hemorrhage at the arterial puncture site or, less frequently, thrombosis at this site. Cardiac arrhythmias and conduction abnormalities may occur during the study and are usually transient and do not require any specific treatment, although ventricular tachycardia and fibrillation are possible.

Although coronary arteriography is still considered the definitive test for coronary artery disease, it also has its limitations. Because the angiograms are interpreted visually, there are often differences in interpretation of the severity of a specific lesion, particularly when the lesion is not seen equally well in various views. It is not uncommon, therefore, for one angiographer to interpret a lesion as significant, and another angiographer to interpret the same lesion as insignificant, especially when the lesion is in the 50-70% range of narrowing.

Another limitation which must be borne in mind is that coronary arteriography reveals only anatomy and not physiology. The demonstration of one or more significant coronary lesions does not necessarily establish a causal relationship with a patient's symptoms or predict with accuracy the patient's prognosis.

REFERENCES

Conti, C. R.: Coronary arteriography, in Weissler, A. M. (Ed.), "Reviews of Contemporary Laboratory Methods," American Heart Association, Dallas, 1980, pp. 129.

Conti, C. R., Levin, D. C., and Grossman, W.: Coronary angiography, in Grossman, W. (Ed.), "Cardiac Catheterization and Angiography," Lea & Febiger, Philadelphia, 1980, pp. 147-169.

Davis, K. , Kennedy, J. W. , Kemp, H. G. , Judkins, M. P. ,
Gosselin, A. J. , and Killip, T. : Complications of coronary
arteriography from the collaborative study of coronary artery
surgery (Cass).   Circulation 59, 1979, pp. 1105-1124.

Franch, R. H. , King, S. B. , III, and Douglas, J. W. : Techniques of cardiac catheterization including coronary arteriography, in Hurst, J. W. (Ed.), "The Heart," McGraw-Hill,
New York, 1982, pp. 1843-1880.

Gensini, G. C. : Coronary arteriography, in Braunwald, E.
(Ed.), "Heart Disease," W. B. Saunders, Philadelphia, 1980,
pp. 308-360.

Hempler, F. A. , Proudfit, W. L. , Razavi, M. , Shirey, E. K. ,
Greenstreet, R. , and Sheldon, W. C. : Ergonovine maleate
provocative test for coronary arterial spasm.   Am J Cardiol
41, 1978, 631-640.

Chapter 7

ANGINA PECTORIS—MEDICAL MANAGEMENT

INTRODUCTION

Angina pectoris, as defined in Chapter 2, can be subdivided
into two major types: (1) chronic, stable angina pectoris and
(2) unstable angina pectoris. Although there is frequently an
overlap between these, and patients may progress back and
forth to one form to the other, it is useful to separate them for
the purpose of discussion of management.

STABLE ANGINA PECTORIS

Stable angina pectoris is defined as angina which is not changing
in any of its characteristics (frequency, severity, duration, or
ease of provocation). Since angina pectoris is a result of an
imbalance between myocardial oxygen supply (due to diseased
coronary arteries) and myocardial oxygen demand, the treatment of angina pectoris depends entirely upon increasing the
oxygen supply and decreasing the oxygen demand. In general,
stable angina pectoris is due to fixed (as contrasted with
spastic) coronary lesions, and, therefore, medical treatment
of this disorder must depend upon reduction of myocardial
oxygen demand rather than on an increase in oxygen blood supply. The major determinants of myocardial oxygen demand
are heart rate, systolic blood pressure ("afterload"), and left
ventricular size ("preload"). The first step toward treatment
of angina is to identify any reversible factors which may be
contributing to an increase of any of these determinants:

1. Hypertension
2. Resting and/or Exercise Tachycardia
3. Heart Failure
4. Emotional or Physical Stress

Hypertension should be treated with appropriate drugs (drugs
which result in reflex tachycardia should generally not be used
without addition of beta-blocking drugs). Heart failure should be

treated with diuretics and digitalis. A resting tachycardia may indicate congestive heart failure or poor physical conditioning and will result in an exaggerated heart rate response to exercise which will thereby lower the threshold of exercise-induced angina pectoris. Physical conditioning by means of an appropriate exercise program (see Chapter 9 on Cardiac Rehabilitation) will help to reduce both resting and exercise heart rates. Avoidance of emotionally and physically stressful situations should be emphasized. Sudden isometric forms of exercise should especially be eliminated. Agents which increase heart rate and/or blood pressure, such as cigarettes and stimulants, should be avoided or curtailed.

In the initial evaluation as well as subsequent periodic reevaluation, an exercise test (bicycle or treadmill) should be performed to establish the exercise level, heart rate, and blood pressure at which angina pectoris is produced to establish a baseline for therapy as well as to determine recommendations for exercise. In addition, the exercise test will help to separate those patients with critical coronary disease who may be best treated surgically (aortocoronary bypass) from those who should be managed more conservatively.

DRUG TREATMENT OF ACUTE ATTACKS

The basic pharmacologic therapy for angina pectoris remains the nitrate group of drugs of which nitroglycerin is the standard and primary treatment. Although there continues to be some debate about the mechanism of action of nitroglycerin in relieving angina pectoris, the principal mechanism is probably peripheral venous dilatation and pooling with resultant decrease in left ventricular volume and pressure (decreased preload), thus reducing myocardial oxygen demand. In addition, nitroglycerin reduces systolic arterial pressure by decreased venous return and, to a lesser extent, by some direct arterial vasodilatation (decreased afterload), thus further reducing myocardial oxygen demand. Nitroglycerin also directly dilates coronary arteries and may increase subendocardial blood flow, but in the absence of coronary spasm, it is doubtful that this is a major mechanism in relieving angina.

Nitroglycerin tablets are available in four dose strengths: 0.15 mg (1/400 g), 0.3 mg (1/200 g), 0.4 mg (1/150 g), and 0.6 mg (1/100 g), all of which are sublingual. Generally, patients are started on one of the intermediate dosage strengths and then either titrated up or down according to response and side effects (headache, flushing, tachycardia, dizziness, or light-headedness). The patient who is not accustomed to taking nitroglycerin should be advised to sit or lie down prior to placing the tablet under the tongue to avoid orthostatic hypotension. Ordinarily, relief of an attack of angina pectoris should occur within 1 to 2 minutes of taking the nitroglycerin (assuming the tablet is fresh). If relief is not complete within 5-10 minutes, the patient should repeat the dose once or twice more, leaving 10-15 minutes between doses until a maximum of three doses has been taken. Failure to obtain relief within three doses in a 30-45-minute period usually indicates either that the chest pain represents an episode of coronary insufficiency or acute myocardial infarction or that it is noncardiac pain. In order to avoid stale and ineffective nitroglycerin tablets, the tablets should be stored in a dark and cool area, and once opened the bottle should be discarded after 3 months. Alternatively, a stabilized preparation (Nitrostat) may be used which has a much longer shelf life and is particularly useful for patients with infrequent attacks of angina pectoris.

In addition to sublingual nitroglycerin, several other forms of nitrates can be used to abort an acute attack of angina pectoris, including inhaled amyl nitrite (which is slightly faster than sublingual nitroglycerin but causes more arterial dilatation and hypotension) and other sublingual and chewable forms of nitrate (Table 7-1) which take slightly longer to work but have a longer duration of action. Many patients find that it is not necessary to take nitroglycerin to abort attacks of exercise-induced angina pectoris, and instead either rest for a few minutes until the attack subsides, or (in some cases) continue their activity with spontaneous subsidence of the pain ("walk-through angina"). Some patients find that the side effects of nitroglycerin are more unpleasant than a mild attack of angina and prefer to allow the attack to subside spontaneously rather than using nitroglycerin.

PREVENTATIVE TREATMENT OF ANGINA

1. Nitrates

Since it is generally preferable to prevent attacks of angina pectoris rather than treat acute attacks, preventative (prophylactic) treatment represents the major pharmacologic approach to this condition. Nitrates, both in long- and short-acting forms also form the mainstay of preventative medical treatment. Ordinary sublingual nitroglycerin is highly effective in preventing attacks of angina pectoris when taken immediately prior to activity, and many patients rely on this form of prophylaxis. In other patients in whom the initiation of anginal attacks is less predictable (or more frequent), longer-acting forms of nitro-glycerin are preferable. Many forms, dosages, and brands of long-acting nitrates are on the market, all of which are effective, and the choice is usually determined by patient or physician preferences (Table 7-1). The correct dose of any of these drugs varies with the individual patient and must be titrated to find the dose that is most effective in preventing angina and least productive of side effects.

Side Effects

Hypotension, headaches, dizziness, flushing, nausea.

Contraindications to Nitrate Therapy

The only strict contraindications to nitrate use is the presence of significant hypotension. Although many patients may develop orthostatic hypotension with nitrate therapy, it is usually possible to reduce the dosage to the point where this no longer occurs.

2. Beta-Adrenergic Blocker Therapy

Along with nitrates, the group of drugs known as beta-adrenergic blocking agents forms the other standard pharmacologic basis of preventative therapy of angina pectoris. This group of drugs reduces myocardial oxygen demand by a number of mechanisms including reduction of heart rate, reduction of systolic blood pressure, and decrease in the force and rate of myocardial contraction. In general, a combination of a nitrate and a beta-blocker is a highly effective preventative form of therapy. As with the nitrates, a variety of individual drugs are available, and the dosage of any given drug varies with the individual patient, and therapy should be individualized (Table 7-2). The drug which has been in longest use in this country and is still the standard drug in this class is propranolol (Inderal). Some of the newer drugs have the advantages of being cardiac (beta-1) selective (in lower dosages), which is an advantage in treating patients with obstructive pulmonary disease, diabetes mellitus, and peripheral vascular disease, and some of the newer drugs have a longer duration of action. One drug (pindolol) has the unique property of intrinsic sympathomimetic activity, which may allow its use in patients with resting bradycardia or mildly impaired cardiac function. As of this time, although all beta-blocking drugs are theoretically useful in angina pectoris, only propranolol (Inderal) and nadolol (Corgard) have been approved for this specific application in this country.

Table 7-1. Nitrate Drugs

Route of Administration	Generic Name	Brand Names	Dosage Strengths	Usual Dosages	Onset of Action	Duration of Action
Sublingual	Nitroglycerin (Glyceryl Trinitrate)	Nitrostat	0.15, 0.3, 0.4, 0.6 mg	0.3 or 0.4 mg prn up to q 15 min x 3	30 sec	20-30 min
	Isosorbide dinitrate	Isordil Sorbitrate	2.5, 5, 10 mg	2.5 to 10 mg q 3-4 hr	2-5 min	2-4 hr
	Erythrityl tetranitrate	Cardilate	5, 10, 15 mg	10 mg prn to 100 mg/day	5 min	2 hr
Transmucosal (Buccal)	Nitroglycerin	Susadrin	1 and 2 mg	1-2 t.i.d. or q.i.d.	3 min	5-6 hr
Chewable	Isosorbide dinitrate	Isordil Sorbitrate	5 and 10 mg	5 or 10 mg q 3-4 hr	5 min	2-4 hr
	Erythrityl tetranitrate	Cardilate	10 mg	10 mg q 3-4 hr	5 min	2-4 hr
Oral	Nitroglycerin (Sustained Release)	Nitrobid Nitrostat Nitrospan Nitrong Nitroglyn	1.3, 2.5, 2.6, 6.5, 9 mg	2.5-9 mg q 8-12 hr	20-30 min	8-12 hr

Isosorbide dinitrate	Isordil Sorbitrate Dilatrate-SR	5, 10, 20, 30, 40 mg, and 40 mg SA	10-40 mg q 6 hr 40 mg q 8-12 hr	15-30 min 15-30 min	4-6 hr 8-12 hr
Erythrityl tetranitrate	Cardilate	5, 10, 15 mg	10 mg q 4-6 hr	30 min	4-6 hr
Pentaery-thritol tetranitrate	Peritrate	10, 20, 40 mg, and 80 mg SA	10-20 mg q 4-6 hr 80 mg q 8-12 hr	20 min 20 min	4-6 hr 8-12 hr
Nitroglycerin (ointment)	Nitrol Nitrobid Nitrostat	2%	1/2-2 inches q 4-8 hr	15-30 min	4-8 hr
Transdermal (Topical) Nitroglycerin (patch)	Nitrodur	5, 10, 15, 20 cm^2 (26, 51, 77, 104, 154 mg)	10-20 cm^2 q 24 hr	30 min	24 hr
	Nitrodisc	5, 10 mg/24 hr (16 mg, 32 mg content)	5-10 mg q 24 hr	30 min	24 hr
	Transderm-Nitro	2.5, 5, 10, 15 mg/24 hr (12.5, 25, 50, 75 mg content)	5-10 mg q 24 hr	30 min	24 hr

Table 7-2.   Beta-Adrenergic Drugs

Generic Name	Brand Name	Dosage Strengths	Usual Dose Ranges
I. Nonselective Drugs (β 1 and β 2)			
Propranolol	Inderal (Inderal LA)	10, 20, 40, 60, 80, 90 mg 80, 120, 160 mg	20-80 mg t.i.d.-q.i.d. 80-320 mg once daily
Nadolol	Corgard	40 and 80 mg	40-240 mg once daily
*Timolol	Blockadren	5 and 10 mg	10-30 mg b.i.d.
* † Pindolol	Visken	5 and 10 mg	5-10 mg b.i.d.
II. Cardiac (β 1) Selective Drugs			
*Metoprolol	Lopressor	50 and 100 mg	25-200 mg b.i.d. (or 100-200 mg once daily)
*Atenolol	Tenormin	50 mg	50-200 mg once daily

*Not yet approved for treatment of angina pectoris
† Has intrinsic sympathomimetic activity

Generally, when first starting a patient on one of these drugs, a fairly low dose is used (for example, 10-20 mg of propranolol, three to four times per day), particularly if the patient is not hospitalized, or has bradycardia, low blood pressure, is elderly, or has borderline cardiac function or an enlarged heart. Once it is determined that the initial dose is well tolerated (there is no excessive bradycardia or hypotension or development of congestive heart failure or bronchospasm), the dose can be gradually increased until an adequate therapeutic effect is observed. Usually the heart rate as well as the clinical response is used as a guide to achieving the effective dose, with a therapeutic range of resting heart rate usually being 55-65 beats per minute. When starting a normotensive patient on a beta-blocker drug for the first time as an outpatient, it is often advisable not to start it simultaneously with a nitrate, in case the combined effects produce an exaggerated hypotensive response. Whenever feasible, therefore, several days should elapse between the initiation of these two types of drugs when used together. In addition to the synergistic effect of reducing myocardial oxygen demand when both of these drugs are used together, their combined use has the advantage of blocking the reflex tachycardia often seen when nitrates are used alone. A note of warning in the use of beta-blocking drugs pertains to the acute withdrawal syndrome seen when there is sudden discontinuation of drug therapy, particularly when the dose is high. Acceleration of angina, development of unstable angina pectoris, and even acute myocardial infarction and sudden death can occur in this setting. Patients should therefore be warned of this and advised not to discontinue therapy on their own. If it is necessary to discontinue beta-blocker therapy, the dose should be gradually reduced prior to discontinuation.

Side Effects

Bradycardia, hypotension, bronchial constriction, congestive heart failure, heart block, cool extremities, tiredness, depression, impotence, alopecia, diarrhea, and interference with response to hypoglycemia.

Contraindications

The only strict contraindications to the use of beta-blocking drugs are marked bradycardia (resting heart rate less than 50), sick sinus syndrome, second degree A-V heart block, significant congestive heart failure, and Raynaud's disease or phenomenon. Beta-blockers can be used with caution in patients with mild bradycardia (rates 50-60), first degree A-V block, mild or compensated congestive heart failure, and in patients with low-normal blood pressure (systolic blood pressure of 95-110). Cardiac selective beta-blocking drugs (or pindolol) can be used with caution in patients with obstructive lung disease, diabetes mellitus, and peripheral vascular disease, but these patients must be watched closely, using the lowest possible effective dose of these drugs.

3.   Calcium Channel Blocking Drugs

This is the newest class of drugs applicable to the preventative treatment of angina pectoris. Although initially felt to be indicated only in patients with coronary spasm (see below), it has been well demonstrated that this group of drugs, used alone or more commonly in conjunction with nitrates and/or beta-blockers, is also an effective form of therapy for exertional angina. The mechanisms of action include a combination of afterload reduction (arterial dilatation) and direct coronary artery dilatation and prevention of coronary arterial spasm. In addition, verapamil (and to lesser extent, diltiazem) decrease cardiac contractility. Although the basic mechanism of all these drugs is the same, their relative effects on arterial pressure, myocardial contractility, heart rate, and conduction differ (Table 7-3).

At the present time, calcium blocking drugs are generally used for treating stable angina pectoris only after failure of nitrates and beta-blockers to control angina symptoms. In some cases, however, the calcium blocking drugs can be used to substitute for either a nitrate or beta-blocker if the patient is unable to tolerate either of these classes of drugs. In most cases, the calcium blockers are used in addition to a nitrate and/or beta-blocker for refractory cases of angina pectoris. All three currently available calcium blockers appear to be equally effective in preventing exertional angina. However, there are differences: nifedipine tends to be associated with more frequent side effects than verapamil due to greater vasodilatation and reflex tachycardia, while verapamil should not be the drug of choice in patients with abnormal cardiac function or with bradycardia or A-V conduction abnormalities. Diltiazem is associated with the lowest incidence of side effects and may therefore be a good choice for initial calcium blocker treatment of angina pectoris.

Table 7-3.   Calcium Channel Blocking Drugs

Generic Name	Brand Names	Dosage Strengths	Usual Dose Range	Effects on				
				Blood Pressure	Heart Rate	A-V Conduction	Contractile Force	Coronary Dilatation
Nifedipine	Procardia	10, 20 mg	10–40 mg t.i.d.–q.i.d.	↓↓↓	↑	0	0	↑↑↑
Verapamil	Calan, Isoptin	80, 120 mg	80–120 mg t.i.d.–q.i.d.	↓↓	-↑↓	↓↓↓ / ↓↓↓ -	↓↓ / ↓↓	↑ / ↑
Diltiazem	Cardizem	30, 60 mg	30–60 mg q.i.d.	↓	0 -↓	↓↓ / ↓	0 -↓	↑↑↑

The direction and number of arrows indicate the type (increase or decrease) and magnitude of effect.
O = No effect.

Side Effects

The most common side effects are dizziness, light-headedness, flushing, headaches, palpitations, nausea, constipation, and peripheral edema. In general, these adverse reactions respond to decreasing the dosage or to continued use. It should be noted that digoxin levels are increased when these drugs are used in conjunction with digitalis drugs.

Contraindications

Verapamil is contraindicated in patients with congestive heart failure and with SA or AV nodal conduction abnormalities, and should generally not be used in conjunction with other drugs with negative inotropic effects (beta-blockers or disopyromide [Norpace]). Because they lower blood pressure, all three drugs should be used with caution in patients with borderline to low blood pressure and in patients with hepatic or renal dysfunction.

GENERAL PLAN OF PHARMACOLOGIC THERAPY OF STABLE ANGINA PECTORIS

Figure 7-1 illustrates the general scheme of pharmacologic approach to the treatment of stable angina pectoris. Although either a nitrate or beta-blocker can be used as the initial drug in the treatment of angina pectoris, individual patient characteristics often determine which drug is preferred. Patients with hypertension or tachycardia are ideally suited for beta-blockers, while patients with relative or absolute contraindications to beta-blocker therapy should be started on nitrate therapy.

UNSTABLE ANGINA PECTORIS

Unstable angina pectoris refers to a change in the course of stable angina pectoris in that there is an increase in the frequency, severity, duration, and/or ease of provocation. An episode (or episodes) of angina occurring at rest associated with increased duration or intensity is also referred to as preinfarction angina, rest angina, coronary insufficiency, angina decubitus, or the intermediate coronary syndrome. The occurrence or development of this syndrome in patients with or without prior stable angina pectoris is usually associated with severe coronary artery disease and often results in subsequent myocardial infarction or continued and progressive angina

INITIATE TREATMENT WITH:

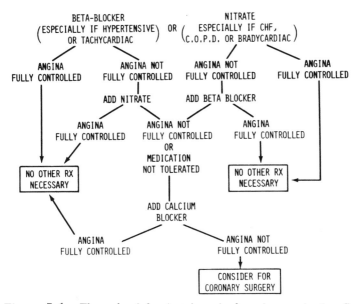

Figure 7-1. Flow chart for treatment of angina pectoris. See text for discussion. (CHF = congestive heart failure, C.O.P.D. = chronic obstructive pulmonary disease, RX = treatment)

pectoris. Such patients also tend to have more rapid progression of coronary atherosclerosis. In at least some cases, rest angina pectoris may be partially a result of coronary artery spasm (or increased coronary artery tone) in addition to fixed coronary artery disease.

Patients with stable angina pectoris who manifest a slight to moderate increase in angina ("progressive" or "crescendo" angina) should have their therapy reviewed and optimized, as discussed in the above section on stable angina pectoris. Patients who do not respond to an increase in medical therapy should undergo coronary arteriography for delineation of coronary anatomy and consideration for coronary bypass surgery or angioplasty.

Patients with a marked increase in their anginal pattern and patients with rest angina should, in general, be hospitalized in a monitored unit and observed closely. Activities should initially consist of bed rest with limited bathroom privileges, and oxygen and sedatives should be used as necessary. Obvious contributing factors should be eliminated or treated (smoking, emotional and physical stress, hypertension, heart failure, or arrhythmias) and medication (nitrates and beta-blockers) should be increased until symptoms are relieved or tolerance is exceeded (side effects or excessive bradycardia or hypotension).

If these steps fail to adequately control the episodes of angina, other medical modalities should be tried, which would include the addition of a calcium channel blocker (particularly if coronary spasm is suspected) and/or the use of intravenous nitroglycerin. Intravenous nitroglycerin is a powerful venous and arterial dilator and requires close monitoring of blood pressure and volume status and is best done with arterial and pulmonary artery (Swan-Ganz) catheters for continuous hemodynamic assessment, although it can be used with frequent blood pressure determination (with an automated device) alone. The dose of a continuous drip of intravenous nitroglycerin must be tailored to the individual patient according to clinical response and arterial pressure. A usual starting dose is 5-10 $\mu g/min$ which is increased every 3-5 minutes by 5-10 μg until the acute episode of pain is relieved or until arterial blood pressure falls by 20 mmHg from a previous normal blood pressure, or to a normal pressure if the patient is hypertensive. The patient is maintained on this continuous drip until stable, and the dose is then titrated down gradually in an attempt to switch back to an oral, sublingual, or topical form of nitrate.

Although anticoagulant and platelet inhibiting drugs have been advocated for the treatment of unstable angina pectoris for years, the recent Veterans Administration Cooperative Study has just recently clearly established the safety and significant effect of low-dose (324 mg) aspirin on reducing the incidence of acute myocardial infarction and death (in men). It would therefore appear that this should be an early and important part of the routine treatment of unstable angina pectoris. (In patients unable to tolerate aspirin, dipyridamole (Persantine) or sulfinpyrazone (Anturane) might be suitable alternatives.) One potential disadvantage to using aspirin routinely is that bleeding time may be prolonged for up to a week, and this may potentially interfere with cardiac catheterization or coronary bypass surgery done within this time and may require correction with platelet transfusions if either of these procedures is required emergently. Alternatively, a heparin infusion (or even streptokinase) may be effective, since intermittent intracoronary thrombosis may be the mechanism of some cases of rest angina.

In the rare patient who cannot be controlled with any medical regimen, it may be necessary to use intraarterial balloon counterpulsation (see Chapter 8) to eliminate episodes of severe rest angina.

Patients who respond easily to medical therapy can gradually be ambulated and either discharged or subjected to coronary arteriography prior to discharge. The timing of arteriography in this group of patients should be related to the necessity and timing of anticipated coronary bypass surgery, and in general it is now felt that there is less of a consistent and emergent need for this approach. The group of patients who respond to medical therapy can be followed as outpatients over the next few weeks and months and often return to their previous level of stable angina pectoris without increased infarction rate or mortality. Noninvasive testing (treadmill and/or nuclear stress test) should generally be performed when these patients are stabilized to assess their status. Coronary arteriography can be performed electively if indicated by continued clinical symptomatology or by significant abnormalities on noninvasive testing. If a progressive angina pattern recurs, angiography and consideration of surgery or angioplasty should then be planned.

Patients who require continued intravenous nitroglycerin and/or intraaortic balloon counterpulsation or do not respond completely to medical therapy should have coronary arteriography performed during their hospitalization, and surgery should be performed in suitable patients. Some of these patients may be candidates for a newer form of invasive therapy, percutaneous transluminal coronary angioplasty (PTCA), discussed in Chapter 10.

VARIANT ANGINA ("PRINZMETAL'S ANGINA")

This relatively uncommon form of angina pectoris is characterized by angina at rest and by ST segment elevation rather than depression during episodes of pain. Episodes are often associated with ventricular arrhythmias and/or A-V block. This syndrome is usually caused by coronary artery spasm, with or without associated arteriosclerotic coronary artery disease. Suspected cases of coronary spasm who do not have observed episodes of ST segment elevation with pain can often be diagnosed by intravenous injection of ergonovine maleate during coronary arteriography, which produces coronary spasm in patients who are subject to this condition (Figure 6-4.)

The acute episodes of pain usually respond to nitroglycerin, and attacks can often be prevented by the use of long-acting nitrates. The recent availability of calcium channel blocking drugs, however, has resulted in a vast improvement in the preventative treatment of this syndrome, since these drugs are effective in preventing coronary spasm. In general, beta-blocking drugs should not be used, since they tend to have an

adverse effect on coronary vasodilatation and cause an increase in angina. Patients who do not respond satisfactorily to treatment with calcium blocking drugs should undergo coronary arteriography to identify those with superimposed or severe arteriosclerotic coronary artery lesions who may be candidates for coronary bypass surgery.

REFERENCES

ANGINA PECTORIS—GENERAL PRINCIPLES

Amsterdam, E. A.: Optimal medical therapy for angina pectoris. Pract Cardiol 8, 1982, pp. 41-45.

Cohn, P. F. and Braunwald, E.: Chronic coronary artery disease, in Braunwald, E. (Ed.), "Heart Disease," W. B. Saunders, Philadelphia, 1980, pp. 1387-1436.

Reeves, T. J.: Medical management of the patient with angina pectoris: An overview of the problem. Circulation 65 (Suppl. II), 1982, II-3-II-13.

Sonnenblick, E. H.: Step-care therapy in the treatment of ischemic heart disease. Cardiovasc Rev 3, 1982, pp. 1283-1289.

UNSTABLE ANGINA—GENERAL PRINCIPLES

Hultgren, H. N., Shetligar, U. R., and Miller, C.: Medical vs. surgical treatment of unstable angina. Am J Cardiol 50, 1982, pp. 663-670.

Lewis, H. D., Jr., et al.: Protective effects of aspirin against acute myocardial infarction and death in men with unstable angina. Results of a Veterans Administration Cooperative Study. N Engl J Med 309, 1983, pp. 396-403.

Moise, A., Theroux, P., Theymans, Y., Descoings, B., Lesperance, J., Waters, D. D., Pelletier, G. B., and Bourassa, M. G.: Unstable angina and progression of coronary atherosclerosis. N Engl J Med 309, 1983, pp. 685-689.

Mulcahy, R., Daly, L., Graham, I., Hickey, N., O'Donoghue, S., Owens, A., Ruane, P., and Tobin, G.: Unstable angina: Natural history and determinants of prognosis. Am J Cardiol 48, 1981, pp. 525-528.

Oliva, P. B. : Unstable rest angina with ST segment depression. Ann Intern Med 100, 1984, pp. 424-440.

Rackley, C. E. , Russell, R. O. , Rogers, W. J. , Mantle, J. A. , and Papapietro, S. E. : Unstable angina pectoris: Is it time to change our approach? Am Heart J 103, 1982, pp. 154-156.

Russell, R. O. , Rackley, C. E. , and Kouchoukos, N. T. : Unstable angina pectoris: Management based on available information. Circulation 65 (Suppl II), 1982, II-72-II-77.

VARIANT ANGINA AND CORONARY SPASM

Conti, C. R. , Feldman, R. L. , and Pepine, C. J. : Coronary artery spasm: Prevalence, clinical significance, and provocative testing. Am Heart J 103, 1982, pp. 584-588.

Ginsburg, R. , Schroeder, J. S. , and Harrison, D. C. : Coronary artery spasm. Pathophysiology, clinical presentations, diagnostic approaches and rational treatment. West J Med 136, 1982, pp. 398-410.

Gorlin, R. : Role of coronary vasospasm in the pathogenesis of myocardial ischemia and angina pectoris. Am Heart J 103, 1982, pp. 598-603.

Maseri, A. , Severi, S. , DeNes, M. , L'abbate, A. , Chierchia, S. , Marzilli, M. , Ballestra, A. M. , Parodi, O. , Biagini, A. , and Distante, A. : "Variant" angina: One aspect of a continuous spectrum of vasospastic myocardium ischemia. Am J Cardiol 42, 1978, pp. 1019-1035.

Schroeder, J. S. , Rosenthal, S. , Ginsburg, R. , and Lamb, I. : Medical therapy of variant angina. Chest 78 (Suppl.), 1980, pp. 231-233.

NITRATE DRUGS

Abrams, J. : Nitroglycerin and long-acting nitrates in clinical practice. Am J Med 74, 1983, pp. 85-94.

Aronow, W. S. : Clinical use of nitrates. 1. Nitrates as anti-anginal drugs. Mod Conc Cardiovasc Dis 48, 1979, pp. 31-35.

Feldman, R. L. and Conti, C. R. : Relief of myocardial
ischemia with nitroglycerin: What is the mechanism? Circulation 64, 1981, pp. 1098-1100.

McGregor, M. : Pathogenesis of angina pectoris and role of
nitrates in relief of myocardial ischemia. Am J Med 74,
6/27/83, pp. 21-27.

Mikolich, J. R. , Nicoloff, N. B. , Robinson, P. H. , and
Logue, R. B. : Relief of refractory angina with continuous
intravenous infusion of nitroglycerin. Chest 77, 1980, pp.
375-379.

Reichek, N. : Role of nitroglycerin in effort angina. Am J
Med 74, 6/27/83, pp. 33-39.

Russell, R. O. , Jr. : Nitrates in the treatment of angina
pectoris. Cardiovasc Rev Rep 5, 1984, pp. 15-25.

Scheidt, S. S. : Nitrates in angina - a classic drug revisited.
Cardiovasc Rev Rep 5, 1984, pp. 45-53.

BETA-ADRENERGIC BLOCKING DRUGS

Frishman, W. H. : B-adrenoceptor antagonists: New drugs and
new indications. N Engl J Med 305, 1981, pp. 500-506.

Frishman, W. H. : Nadolol: A new beta-adrenoceptor antagonist. N Engl J Med 305, 1981, pp. 678-682.

Frishman, W. H. : Atenolol and timolol, two new systemic β
adrenoceptor antagonists. N Engl J Med 306, 1982, pp. 1456-1462.

Jackson, G. : Comparative efficacy and safety of beta-blockers
in angina pectoris. Primary Cardiol 1 (Suppl 1), 1980, pp.
97-101.

Kostis, J. B. , Frishman, W. , Hosler, M. H. , Thorsen, N. L. ,
Gonasun, L. , and Weinstein, J. : Treatment of angina pectoris
with pindolol: The significance of intrinsic sympathomimetic
activity of beta-blockers. Am Heart J 104, 1982, pp. 496-504.

Rogers, W. J. : Use of beta blockers in the treatment of
ischemic heart disease: A comparison of the available agents.
Cardiovasc Rev Rep 5, 1984, pp. 31-43.

CALCIUM CHANNEL BLOCKING DRUGS

Dawson, J. R. , Whitaker, N. H. G. , and Sutton, G. C. :
Calcium antagonist drugs in chronic stable angina. Comparison of verapamil and nifedipine. Br Heart J 46, 1981, pp. 508-
512.

Gerstenblith, G. , Ouyang, P. , Aschuff, S. C. , Bulkey, B. H. ,
Becker, L. C. , Mellits, E. D. , Baughman, K. L. , Weiss,
J. L. , Flaherty, J. T. , Kallman, C. H. , Llewellyn, M. , and
Weisfeldt, M. : Nifedipine in unstable angina. A double-blind,
randomized trial. N Engl J Med 306, 1982, pp. 885-889.

Henry, P. D. : Comparative pharmacology of calcium antagonists: Nifedipine, verapamil and diltiazem. Am J Cardiol 46,
1980, pp. 1047-1058.

Frishman, W. H. , Klein, N. A. , Strom, J. A. , Willens, H. ,
Lejemtel, T. H. , Jentzer, J. , Siegel, L. , Klein, P. , Kirschen,
N. , Silverman, R. , Pollock, S. , Doyle, R. , Kirsten, E. , and
Sonnenblick, E. : Superiority of verapamil to propranolol in
stable angina pectoris: A double-blind, randomized crossover
trial. Circulation 65 (Suppl. 1), 1982, I-51-I-59.

Hossock, K. F. , Pool, P. E. , Steele, P. , Crawford, M. H. ,
DeMaria, A. N. , Cohen, L. S. , and Ports, T. A. : Efficacy
of diltiazem in angina on effort: A multicenter trial. Am J
Cardiol 49, 1982, pp. 567-572.

Krikler, D. M. and Rowland, E. : Clinical value of calcium
antagonists in treatment of cardiovascular disorders. J Am
Coll Cardiol 1, 1983, pp. 355-364.

Packer, M. and Frishman, W. H. : Verapamil therapy for
stable and unstable angina pectoris: Calcium channel antagonists in perspective. Am J Cardiol 50, 1982, pp. 881-885.

Rahimtoola, S. H. (Ed.): The calcium channel blockers:
Mechanism of action and role in angina pectoris. Council on
Clinical Cardiology Newsletter 7, 1982, pp. 1-16.

Singh, B. N. : The pharmacology of slow-channel blocking
drugs. Cardiovasc Rev Rep 4, 1983, pp. 179-192.

Nifedipine for angina pectoris.   The Medical Letter 24, 1982, pp. 39-41.

Oral verapamil for angina pectoris.   The Medical Letter 24, 1982, pp. 56-58.

Diltiazem for angina pectoris.   The Medical Letter 25, 1983, pp. 17-18.

Chapter 8

ACUTE MYOCARDIAL INFARCTION

DIAGNOSIS AND CHARACTERIZATION

Acute myocardial infarction can occur anytime in the temporal
spectrum of ischemic artery disease: it can be the initial clinical manifestation of coronary disease, or it can occur after
years of stable angina pectoris, or it can present as sudden
death, with or without prior clinical indications of coronary
artery disease. In almost all cases the acute event occurs as
the result of sudden thrombotic occlusion of a coronary artery,
usually in the setting of significant arteriosclerotic coronary
artery disease in one or more arteries. In most cases it is a
dramatic event, with severe chest pain and other symptoms,
but in other cases the symptoms may be mild, atypical, or
even absent. A "typical" presentation consists of severe chest
pressure, often with radiation to the arms, throat, jaw, and/or
back. There is frequently accompanying nausea (especially
with inferior wall myocardial infarction), diaphoresis, and
weakness.

PHYSICAL FINDINGS

Physical examination often discloses an anxious, pale, and
diaphoretic patient, but like the history, the examination is also
highly variable, varying from a patient in shock to a patient
with no external signs of cardiovascular compromise. In general, there is some correlation between the physical findings
and the severity of the infarction. A small infarction tends to
produce few if any physical findings, while a large infarction
is much more likely to result in congestive heart failure or
shock. The diagnosis of acute myocardial infarction depends
upon the history, electrocardiogram, and cardiac enzymes
rather than on the physical examination.

77

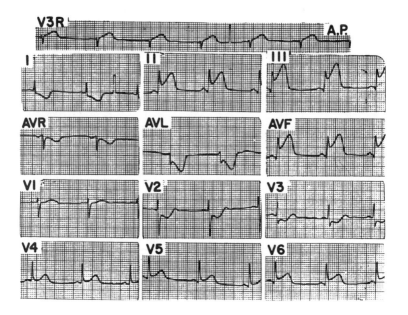

Figure 8-1.   Acute inferoposterior myocardial infarction, illustrating characteristic acute ST elevations in leads II, III, and AVF, with ST depression in leads V_2 and V_3.   Additional ST depressions in leads I and AVL represent reciprocal changes.

ELECTROCARDIOGRAM

The electrocardiogram is still the key to making the diagnosis of acute as well as previous myocardial infarction.   In the first 3 hours of acute infarction, the ECG may not show the characteristic ST and QRS abnormalities that occur later but may show "hyperacute" peaked T waves, or it may be entirely normal.   In acute transmural myocardial infarction, the ST segments typically become elevated in the leads corresponding to the site of infarction, indicative of epicardial injury (leads 2, 3, and AVF for inferior wall infarctions, leads V_1 to V_4 for anteroseptal infarction, and leads 1, AVL and V_5 and V_6 for lateral infarctions).   ST segment depression is seen in leads V_2 to V_4 in true posterior infarction (Figures 8-1, 8-2).   As these ST segment elevations gradually return to normal in the first few days, Q waves develop in the same leads, indicating transmural infarction.   In nontransmural (subendocardial) infarction, there may be ST segment depression and/or T wave inversions indistinguishable from ischemic changes, rather than ST segment

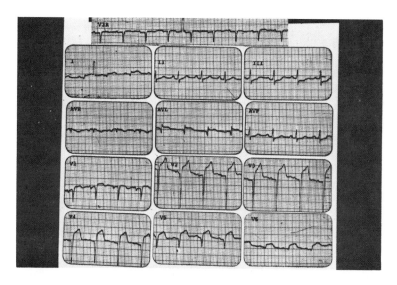

Figure 8-2.   Acute anterior myocardial infarction with additional involvement of the interventricular septum and lateral wall.   There is ST elevation in leads I, AVL, and V_1-V_6.   In addition, Q waves are seen in the same leads.

elevations, and Q waves do not develop (Figures 8-3, 8-4).   In some cases of nontransmural infarction, the electrocardiographic changes may be minimal and nonspecific, and in some cases of small nontransmural infarction, the electrocardiogram may remain normal or unchanged.   It should be kept in mind that the electrocardiogram may be nondiagnostic even with acute transmural myocardial infarction in the presence of complete left bundle branch block, WPW syndrome, ventricular paced rhythm, or prior myocardial infarction in the same anatomic area.

CARDIAC ENZYMES

Equally as important as the electrocardiogram in making the diagnosis of acute myocardial infarction are the cardiac enzymes.   Like the electrocardiogram, the cardiac enzymes also provide information on the acuteness and extent of myocardial infarction, although not the location.   Elevation in creatine kinase (CK) occurs first, appearing in about 6-8 hours after the onset of infarction and peaking in about 18-24 hours.   Of the three isoenzymes of CK (BB, MB, and MM), the MB is myocardial specific, and at least 5% of the total CK found in the

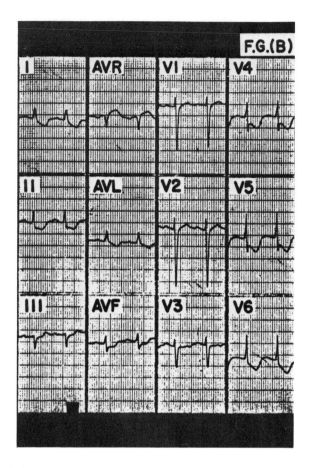

Figure 8-3.   Acute subendocardial infarction illustrating ST depressions in leads I, II, III, AVL, AVF, and V_4-V_6 (inferolateral leads).

blood in acute myocardial infarction is from the MB fraction. CK elevation due entirely to elevations of the MM fraction indicate some source of enzyme release other than the heart and is not consistent with the diagnosis of acute myocardial infarction. Other enzymes which are markers of acute myocardial infarction are the SGOT (AST), which becomes elevated at about 8-12 hours after the onset of acute infarction and peaks at 24-48 hours, and LDH and HBD, which first appear as an increase in the serum level 12-24 hours after the onset of infarction and peak at 2-5 days.   Of the five isoenzymes of LDH, LDH_1 is

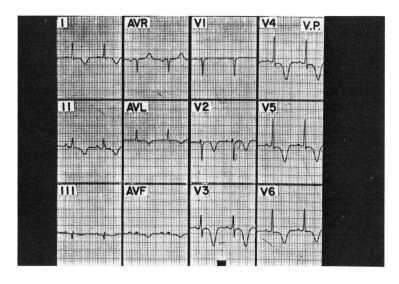

Figure 8-4. Acute subendocardial infarction illustrating T inversions in leads I, II, III, AVL, AVF, and V_2-V_6.

specific for myocardium and red blood cells, and a reversal in the normal LDH_1:LDH_2 ratio so that LDH_1 is greater than LDH_2 is characteristic of acute myocardial infarction. LDH and HBD levels remain elevated longer than the CK and SGOT levels and thus may be helpful in diagnosing infarctions several days after occurrence. In practice, serial cardiac enzymes are obtained on admission and every 8-12 hours for 24 hours, then daily for 3 days in order not to miss small elevations characteristic of small myocardial infarctions and also to determine the peak value of CK, which is proportional to the extent of infarction. If reinfarction is suspected during the course of acute infarction, serial enzymes are reobtained in the same manner.

OTHER INDICATORS OF ACUTE MYOCARDIAL INFARCTION

Although the diagnosis of acute myocardial infarction is usually easily made on the basis of the history, electrocardiograms, and enzymes, the use of other modalities for both diagnosis and characterization is sometimes very helpful, especially in difficult cases.

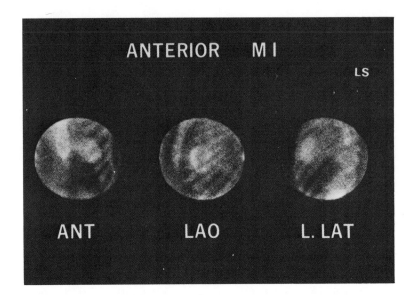

Figure 8-5. Pyrophosphate scan of a patient with an acute anterior myocardial infarction, illustrating a large area of uptake in the heart (to the left of the sternum in the anterior view, posterior to the sternum in the LAO view, and anterior to the spine in the lateral view). In these images, pyrophosphate uptake and bone appear as bright areas. (Courtesy of Dr. Daniel S. Berman)

NUCLEAR METHODS

Acute infarct imaging is possible with technetium 99m pyrophosphate scanning ("hot-spot" imaging), in which the isotope is taken up in the area of infarction and appears as a dark (or bright) area on the scan (Figure 8-5). This test is positive between the second and fifth day after infarction and is useful when the electrocardiogram and enzyme tests are nondiagnostic.

Thallium imaging (thallium 201) is also useful for acute infarct imaging, in which a "cold-spot" appears corresponding to the infarction (Figure 8-6). Thallium scans are also abnormal in the presence of acute ischemia without infarction but tend to normalize (reverse) within 4 hours after an acute ischemic event, whereas the scan tends to remain abnormal in the presence of myocardial infarction (nonreversible defect). Thallium imaging does not differentiate between acute and prior myocardial infarction, however.

Abnormalities in wall motion in the area of the acute myocardial infarction appear very rapidly and remain as the infarct

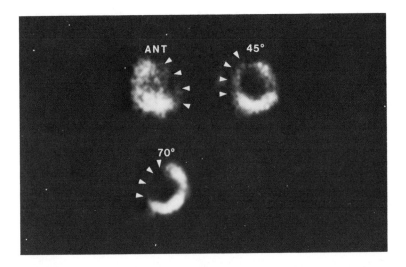

Figure 8-6A. Thallium - 201 imaging in acute myocardial infarction. Anterior (ANT), 45° LAO (45°), and 70° LAD (70°) views in a patient with an acute anteroseptal myocardial infarction (A) and in a patient with an acute inferoposterior myocardial infarction (B). The arrowheads illustrate the regions of decreased or absent thallium uptake. In the patient shown in (A), there is severely reduced uptake in the anterior and septal regions, while in the patient shown in (B), there is severely reduced uptake in the inferior and posterior regions.

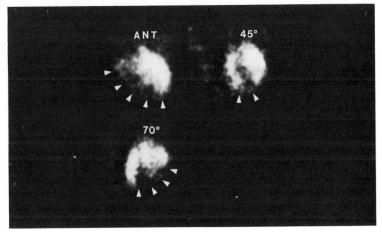

Figure 8-6B.

RIGHT VENTRICULAR INFARCTION

45° LAO

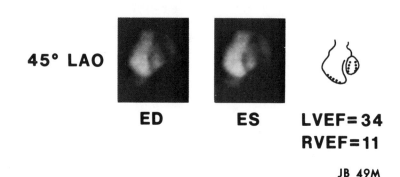

ED   ES   LVEF=34
RVEF=11

JB 49M

Figure 8-7.   Radionuclide ventriculography in a patient with inferoapical myocardial infarction complicated by right ventricular infarction.   The right ventricle is markedly dilated and diffusely hypokinetic, with an ejection fraction of only 11% (contrast this with the normal study shown in Figure 4-3).   (Reproduced by permission, from Berman, D. S. and Mason, D. T. (Eds.), "Clinical Nuclear Cardiology," Grune & Stratton, New York, 1981, p. 273.)

evolves and thus can be demonstrated throughout the course of infarction by radionuclide ventriculography (gated blood pool scintigraphy or first pass scintigraphy) (see Chapter 4).   This technique is most useful in the assessment of the functional significance of acute infarction in that the extent of contraction abnormalities can be easily documented.   It also provides accurate measurement of the left ventricular ejection fraction, which is a good indicator of both immediate and long-term prognosis.   This test is also very useful for diagnosing right ventricular infarction in that it images right ventricular function as well as left ventricular function (Figure 8-7) and can also indicate the presence of mitral regurgitation or ventricular septal rupture.

Two-dimensional echocardiography can also be utilized for determining the presence, location, and extent of myocardial contraction abnormalities associated with acute myocardial infarction of both the left and right ventricles, and like radionuclide ventriculography, serial bedside studies can be performe to provide periodic reassessment.   In addition, two-dimensional echocardiography can be useful for diagnosis of complications of acute infarctions such as pericardial effusion, ventricular septal rupture, mitral regurgitation, and left ventricular aneurysm formation.

MANAGEMENT OF
ACUTE MYOCARDIAL INFARCTION—
GENERAL PRINCIPLES

INITIAL STAGE

The two general goals of managing patients with acute myocardial infarction have traditionally been the control of symptoms and the treatment of complications. More recently, however, another primary goal has been to try to limit the ultimate size of the infarction, and thereby, preventing or decreasing the severity of complications. Although still somewhat investigational, the use of thrombolytic therapy in acute myocardial infarction over the past few years may significantly change the approach to this condition, particularly when the patient is seen within the first few hours of infarction. The subject of limitation of infarct size is discussed later in this chapter. The general guidelines of care remain the same regardless of what time in the course of acute infarction the patient is first seen, and are discussed below.

CARDIAC MONITORING

All patients with acute myocardial infarction should have continuous electrocardiographic monitoring commencing with entrance into the hospital and continued for at least the first 3 days, and longer if arrhythmias or conduction defects develop or there are other major complications.

INTRAVENOUS ACCESS

Upon admission, all patients should have an intravenous catheter placed in an arm vein and maintained patent by a heparin lock. This serves as an access for intravenous medication and is vital in case of an emergency. It is generally maintained for at least the first 3 days or until the patient is stable.

CONTROL OF PAIN

Unlike angina pectoris or coronary insufficiency, the pain of acute myocardial infarction does not usually respond to nitrates but requires potent analgesics. Morphine sulphate remains the most useful agent because of its consistent analgesic effect, rapid onset, its effect in reducing associated anxiety, and the ability to titrate the dose either intravenously or subcutaneously. The major limitations of this drug are the tendency to cause nausea and to produce hypotension and respiratory depression. These complications and side effects can be minimized by avoiding its use in patients with low or borderline blood pressure, by titrating the dose, and by using atropine sulfate if necessary to counteract the vagotonic effects of this drug. A preferred way of administrating morphine sulphate is to give it intravenously 2 mg at a time, checking blood pressure between doses and repeating the dose every 5-10 minutes until pain is relieved or hypotension occurs. If nausea or vomiting occurs it can usually be controlled with antiemetic drugs.

CONTROL OF NAUSEA AND VOMITING

Nausea and vomiting are frequent accompanying symptoms of acute myocardial infarction, especially when it involves the inferior wall of the ventricle. Trimethobenzamide (Tigan) or prochlorperazine (Compazine) can be given intramuscularly, since suppositories may cause a vasovagal reflex bradycardia and hypotension. (The concern about giving intramuscular injections because of resultant elevation of CK levels is not very relevant, since the use of CK isoenzymes easily differentiates between skeletal and myocardial muscle CK.)

ADMINISTRATION OF OXYGEN

Oxygen is administered routinely to patients with acute myocardial infarction, even in the absence of demonstrable hypoxemia. In patients who are not in congestive heart failure and whose arterial oxygen levels are normal, oxygen may be given by nasal cannula at a flow rate of 2-4 liters/min. In patients in congestive heart failure or with hypoxemia, oxygen should be given by mask in higher concentrations and flow rate (unless there is evidence of CO_2 retention).

DIET

There is no specific acute coronary "diet," but general principles do apply:

1. The quantity of food intake should be limited for the first 24 hours because of the frequent development of nausea and vomiting and also to minimize the possibility of aspiration in the event of cardiac arrest due to the

sudden development of arrhythmias or shock.   Furthermore, a light diet reduces the work load of the heart
during this critical first 24-48 hours.

2. There is no need to severely restrict the quantity of
   salt in the diet unless there is evidence of congestive
   heart failure or severe hypertension, but it is a good
   general rule to minimize salt consumption, since heart
   failure at this time may be latent.

3. It is generally advisable to avoid extremely cold and
   extremely hot foods to avoid vagal stimulation.

4. It is advisable to avoid caffeine to avoid myocardial
   stimulation.

5. There is no specific need to place the patient on a low-
   cholesterol and low-fat diet at this stage, although the
   point can be made that this would be a good time to start
   educating the patient as to reduction of these substances.

ACTIVITY

As a general rule, all patients with acute myocardial infarction
should be on strict bed rest for the first 1-2 days, although a
bedside commode is preferable to a bedpan unless the patient
has severe hypotension or shock, pulmonary edema, severe
arrhythmias, or has indwelling catheters for hemodynamic
monitoring. Depending on the state of the patient and the presence or absence of complications, it is generally permissible
as well as beneficial for the patient to get out of bed to sit in a
comfortable chair for short periods after the second or third
hospital day. Discussion of physical activities beyond the first
few hospital days follows later in this chapter.

GENERAL MEDICATION

Medication to be used during the initial few days depends upon individual circumstances, but in general, patients should be on a
stool softener (dioctyl sodium sulfosuccinate or docusate potas-
sium) to reduce the strain of bowel movements. Tranquilizers
are very useful for the anxious patient to avoid tachycardia and
hypertension which may be secondary to stress. However, their
general use is not recommended in the patient who is not particularly anxious.

1. Anticoagulant Drugs

Routine use of anticoagulation (mini-dose, low dose, or full
dose) is not generally recommended in acute myocardial infarction, but individuals at high risk for development of venous

thrombosis should receive mini-dose heparin (5,000-7,500 units subcutaneously Q8-12 hours). Such patients include the elderly, patients who are in congestive heart failure, those anticipated to be on bed rest for more than a few days, those with evidence or history of thrombophlebitis or significant varicose veins, and those with marked obesity. This treatment is continued until the patients are ambulatory.

2. Digitalis

Digitalis is not routinely administered to patients with acute myocardial infarction, including those with congestive heart failure; however, it should be continued in patients who were taking it prior to their acute infarction unless contraindicated (significant bradycardia, heart block, or ventricular arrhythmias).

3. Diuretics

The same principle applies to the use of diuretics: patients who were taking a diuretic prior to their acute infarction for hypertension, congestive heart failure, or edema should generally have this continued unless there is evidence of hypotension or hypovolemia.

4. Nitrates

Nitroglycerin-type drugs are not given routinely to patients with acute myocardial infarction. However, they are also generally continued if patients were on them previously for treatment of angina pectoris unless there is evidence of hypotension or hypovolemia, in which case they should be decreased or, if necessary, stopped. Intravenous nitroglycerin is particularly useful for patients with refractory chest pain, recurrent ischemia, or resistant heart failure (see later discussion).

5. Beta-Blocker Drugs

As discussed in the previous chapter, patients who were chronically taking beta-blocker drugs should never have these drugs withdrawn abruptly. This principle generally applies to patients with acute myocardial infarction who have been maintained on these drugs for treatment of hypertension or angina pectoris. An exception is made, however, if there is severe bradycardia, hypotension, severe congestive heart failure, or significant conduction abnormalities. In patients with milder degrees of these contraindications to continued beta-blocker use, attempts should be made to discontinue the beta-blocker drug gradually rather than suddenly, and this decision must be individualized. This class of drugs can be very useful in patients with inappropriate tachycardia or systolic (and diastolic) hypertension in the absence of any contraindication. The usefulness of beta-blocking drugs to limit infarct size and the role of beta-blocking drugs in prevention of recurrent infarctions and reduction in mortality will be discussed later in this chapter.

6. Antihypertensive Medications

These drugs should generally be continued if taken prior to the infarction, assuming the patient is not hypotensive and there are no contraindications to the continued use of any specific drug.

7. Antiarrhythmic Drugs

These drugs should also generally be continued if the patient was taking one before the acute infarction, except in the presence of severe conduction disturbances, in which case antiarrhythmic drugs are contraindicated. The routine administration of prophylactic antiarrhythmic therapy (usually in the form of lidocaine) to all patients with acute myocardial infarction is still controversial and is generally not recommended when adequate monitoring is available because of the frequent side effects of this drug, particularly in elderly patients and those with congestive heart failure. The use of antiarrhythmic drugs for specific arrhythmias is discussed below.

8. Medications for Limitation of Infarct Size

Over the past several years, a number of pharmacologic agents have been advocated, based on experimental studies, for the therapeutic limitation of infarct size. These agents have included anticoagulants, antiplatelet agents, glucose-insulin-potassium solutions, hyaluronidase, nitrates, calcium channel blocking drugs, and beta-adrenergic blocking drugs. To date, only nitroglycerin (sublingual or intravenous) and the beta-blockers timolol and metoprolol have been shown to have beneficial effects on reducing infarct size and reducing complications when given early in the course of acute infarction. The routine use of these drugs for this purpose is still not clearly established and, therefore, not yet recommended. Recently, a new approach to limiting infarct size has been developed using

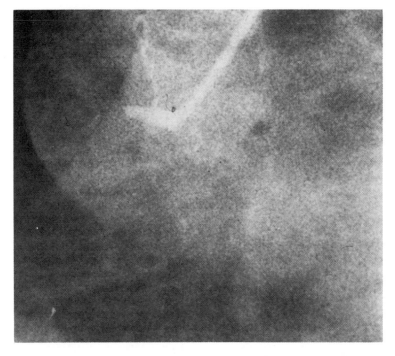

Figure 8-8A. Two frames from a coronary cineangiogram of a
patient with an acute inferior wall myocardial infarction showing
the right coronary artery (LAO view) before (A) and after (B)
direct intracoronary infusion of streptokinase. The initial
angiogram (A) shows complete proximal occlusion of the artery,
while the subsequent angiogram (B) shows a totally patent artery,
but with an area of significant stenosis (arrow) at the site of
prior complete occlusion. (Courtesy of Dr. William Ganz)

thrombolytic agents, which appears effective when applied early
in the course of infarction.

   Thrombolytic Therapy

Acute myocardial infarction appears to be caused in the majority
of cases by thrombosis within a diseased coronary artery. It
has now been shown that the use of an intracoronary injection of
a thrombolytic drug (streptokinase or urokinase) can lyse this
clot and restore effective coronary flow to the infarcted area in
the majority of cases (Figure 8-8). In order for this type of
therapy to effectively limit ultimate infarct size, however, it is

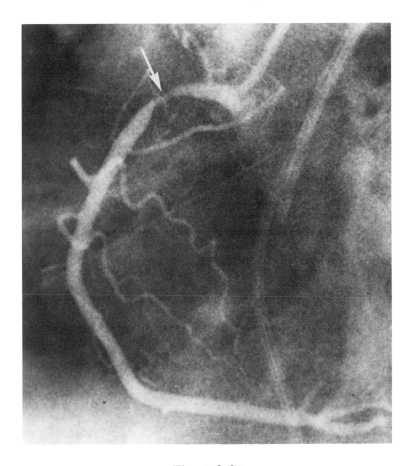

Figure 8-8B.

likely that therapy must be applied in the first 3-4 hours from the onset of the thrombosis (onset of symptoms). At the present time, only direct intracoronary administration of thrombolytic therapy has been approved by the FDA and has been shown to be effective in lysing the clot, increasing myocardial perfusion, improving left ventricular function, and, perhaps, reducing mortality. In this approach it is necessary to insert a special catheter into the thrombosed coronary artery through a standard coronary arteriographic catheter. Although the dose and the method of administration has not been standardized as yet, usually a total dose between 120,000 and 400,000 international units of streptokinase is infused, followed by systemic heparinization

and subsequent use of coumadin for at least 3 months. This
approach obviously requires the availability of a cardiac
catheterization laboratory and team on an emergency basis,
and at the present time, would appear to have limited applica-
bility. This approach should probably be reserved for those
patients who can be treated within the first 3-4 hours of the
onset of infarction and who have had a large infarction with an
anticipated high morbidity and mortality rate. Administration
of streptokinase intravenously (using from 500,000 to 1,500,000
international units) would appear to be a much more applicable
technique for general use and has been shown to reduce the time
to achieve reperfusion from the onset of symptoms by at least
an hour compared to the intracoronary approach. The success
rate of the intravenous approach in thrombolysis has generally
been less than with the intracoronary approach (50% compared
to 75-90%), although a recent study with intravenous streptokinase reported a 96% success rate.

Evidence for clot lysis and reperfusion, in addition to
angiographic and scintigraphic evidence, consists of dramatic
relief of pain, decrease in ST segment elevations (Figure 8-9),
disappearance of conduction disturbances, development of late
ventricular premature beats, and early appearance and peaking
of creatinine kinase in the serum.

The protocol used in the most successful intravenous
streptokinase study involves an initial intravenous bolus of 50-
100 mg of hydrocortisone to prevent allergic reactions, followed
by a 20-minute infusion of 750,000 units of streptokinase in
NaCl, and a repeat dose 20 minutes later, if necessary. This
is followed by I. V. heparin at a dose of 40 units/kg and an infusion of heparin at 15 units/kg/h to keep the PTT $\geq$ 100 seconds.
This is replaced by coumadin after 7 to 10 days for the next 3
months. Serious bleeding (the most frequent complication)
occurs in less than 10% of patients by either route of administration, and the most serious complication (intracerebral
hemorrhage) can be minimized by avoiding streptokinase treatment in patients 75 years or older, especially with diabetes
mellitus, and in patients with severe hypertension or evidence of
cerebrovascular disease. Bleeding complications result because of systemic fibrinolysis and may interfere with invasive
and surgical procedures during the period of fibrinolysis.

The risk of systemic bleeding may be alleviated by two new
developments: tissue plasminogen activator and pro-urokinase.
Both of these agents are naturally occurring substances which
lyse clots without interfering with hemastasis and without the
risk of allergic reaction. Tissue plasminogen activator (T-PA)
can now be obtained by recombinant DNA technology and

ECG CHANGES FOLLOWING REPERFUSION
(VF, 6l y.o., Inf. MI)

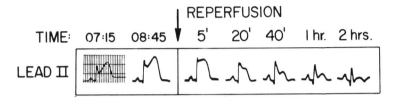

Figure 8-9. ECG changes following reperfusion with streptokinase in a patient with acute inferior wall myocardial infarction
illustrating the rapid decrease in ST segment elevation in lead
II, which was accompanied by rapid relief of chest pain. (Reproduced, with permission, from: Ganz, W., Buchbinder, N.,
Marcus, H., Mondkar, A., Maddahi, J., Charuzi, Y.,
O'Connor, L., Shell, W., Fishbein, M., Kass, R.,
Miyamoto, A., and Swan, H. J. C., Am Heart J 101, 1981,
p. 10.)

pro-urokinase by cell culture, making them practical substitutes
for streptokinase and urokinase. Although initial clinical experience with these agents is limited thus far, their potential
for routine administration in acute myocardial infarction is
exciting, if yet unproven. Although lysis of intracoronary clots
can be easily accomplished and appears to limit infarct size and
improve cardiac performance, the effect on improvement of
immediate and late prognosis is still unsettled, and it is unclear
whether thrombolytic therapy should be applied to all patients
presenting with acute myocardial infarction within the first few
hours of onset of symptoms, or just to a select group of high-
risk patients most likely to benefit from reduction of infarct
size. It is also unclear whether the high-grade coronary lesion
usually seen at the site of intracoronary clot formation should
be managed conservatively or with angioplasty or bypass surgery to prevent reinfarction.

9. Pharmacologic Reduction of Recurrent Myocardial
    Infarction and Mortality

Two pharmacologic approaches have recently been evaluated
with the purpose of prevention of recurrent myocardial infarction

and reduction of postinfarction mortality. One of these involves the use of platelet-inhibiting drugs and the other one the use of beta-adrenergic blocking drugs.

Antiplatelet Drugs

A number of studies have been undertaken to evaluate the effect of antiplatelet drugs (inhibitors of platelet aggregation) on subsequent mortality and reinfarction in patients surviving acute myocardial infarction. Aspirin, sulfinpyrazone (Anturane), and dipyridamole (Persantine) have been tried alone or in combination and have generally shown a trend toward reducing mortality and reinfarction rates, although no definitive results have yet emerged. The dosages and timing of therapy have also not been established.

Beta-Adrenergic Blocking Drugs

Over the past 10 years, 13 major randomized studies involving over 25,000 patients have been conducted to investigate the question of whether long-term treatment with a beta-blocker drug of patients surviving acute myocardial infarction improves survival rate and decreases reinfarction rate. The three largest studies, involving trials with timolol (Norwegian Multicenter Study Groups), propranolol (Beta-Blocker Heart Attack Trial), and metoprolol (Swedish Metoprolol Trial), all showed a significant reduction in mortality of about 35%. These studies have also demonstrated a reduction in death due to cardiovascular causes and to sudden death, as well as a significant reduction in nonfatal recurrent myocardial infarction. The reduction in mortality was most evident in the first 6-12 months, but sustained benefit has been demonstrated for at least 18 months. When patients with contraindications to beta-blocker therapy were excluded (congestive heart failure, bronchial asthma, significant bradycardia or conduction defects, hypotension, or "brittle" diabetes mellitus), the drugs were safe and well tolerated. Although the mechanism of the effect on reduction in mortality and reinfarction is not known, it is postulated to be due to two major mechanisms of the beta-blocker drugs: the antiarrhythmic effects and the antiischemic effects.

At the present time, only two of the beta-blocker drugs have been approved for this "cardiac protective" indication: timolol (Blocadren), at a dose of 10 mg b.i.d., and propranolol (Inderal), at a dose of 60-80 mg t.i.d., although it is felt that other beta-blocker drugs would be expected to have similar effects.

Although it is currently recommended that all patients without contraindications be started on one of these drugs following myocardial infarction, it appears that high-risk patients (especially those with significant arrhythmias and/or left ventricular dysfunction during the acute stage of myocardial infarction) have the most to gain from this approach. It is further recommended that treatment be started from 5 to 10 days after the occurrence of the acute infarction and that it be continued for at least 2 to 3 years.

RECOGNITION AND TREATMENT OF
COMPLICATIONS OF
ACUTE MYOCARDIAL INFARCTION

ARRHYTHMIAS

The major contribution of the CCU has been the reduction of mortality of acute myocardial infarction by control of arrhythmias. All patients with proven or suspected acute myocardial infarction should have constant cardiac monitoring for at least the first 3 days. Although some cardiologists advocate the prophylactic use of intravenous lidocaine in all such patients to prevent the development of ventricular fibrillation, the potential side effects of this drug have made this approach less acceptable than the treatment of arrhythmias as they occur. Although a thorough review of all arrhythmias is beyond the scope of this book, the basic approaches are discussed below.

I. Ventricular Arrhythmias

   A. Ventricular Fibrillation

This arrhythmia is invariably fatal unless treated immediately. A sharp blow to the chest with a closed fist is occasionally effective in terminating this arrhythmia and can be attempted initially, but it is usually necessary to use an electrical defibrillator set at maximum output (400 watt seconds) to terminate ventricular fibrillation. This should be followed by an intravenous bolus of lidocaine (75-100 mg) given immediately following defibrillation and repeated in 10-15 minutes, and a continuous intravenous drip started at a rate of 2 mg/min (and subsequently adjusted at a rate of 1-4 mg/min depending upon clinical response and blood levels). If defibrillation is not immediately successful, it should be reattempted after the initial lidocaine dose has been given.

B.   Ventricular Tachycardia

The approach to the treatment of this arrhythmia depends upon
the ventricular rate as well as the clinical status of the patient.
If the ventricular rate is greater than 150 and/or there is significant hemodynamic compromise observed or the patient suf-
fers loss of consciousness or change in mental status, the
chest thump described above can be tried initially, and if unsuccessful, defibrillation should then be used as described
above.   If the ventricular rate is under 150 and/or there are
no signs of significant hemodynamic compromise or loss of
consciousness, this arrhythmia can be treated pharmacologi-
cally, using a bolus of intravenous lidocaine (75-100 mg)
followed, if successful, by a second bolus and institution of
continuous lidocaine drip.   If lidocaine is ineffective in terminating this arrhythmia, either bretylium tosylate (5 mg/kg by
intravenous bolus) or procainamide (100 mg intravenously
every 5 minutes until effective or a total dose of 1 g is given)
may be tried.   Maintenance bretylium (1-2 mg/min) or procainamide (1-5 mg/min) is then initiated if either of these
agents is successful.   If neither agent is successful in terminating sustained ventricular tachycardia, electrocardioversion
is then indicated.

C.   Slow Ventricular Tachycardia
      (Accelerated Idioventricular Rhythm)

This arrhythmia is commonly seen in the setting of acute myocardial infarction and in contrast to rapid ventricular tachycardia, is a benign arrhythmia.   The rate is usually in the
range of 50-80 and may appear as an escape rhythm in the
setting of sinus bradycardia or as a parasystolic rhythm super-
seding a slower sinus rate.   Since the rate is in a physiologic
range, and the arrhythmia is usually transient, no treatment
is usually necessary, and antiarrhythmic therapy is usually
ineffective.   If the rate is less than 50 and the patient is
symptomatic, treatment with atropine sulfate or temporary
pacing is indicated (see below).

D.   Premature Ventricular Beats
      (PVCs, PVBs, or VPBs)

Because of the lowered fibrillatory threshold in acute myocardial
infarction, the appearance of PVCs in the setting of acute infarction may be preliminary to the development of ventricular
tachycardia or fibrillation and should be treated aggressively

with lidocaine. Patients should receive a bolus of 75-100 mg
(1 mg/kg) intravenously followed by a continuous intravenous
drip of 1-4 mg/min. If the patient is stable and has not developed ventricular tachycardia or ventricular fibrillation after
2 or 3 days on this treatment, the lidocaine can usually be discontinued and the patient observed. Oral antiarrhythmic therapy
can then be initiated with quinidine or procainamide if significant
PVCs recur. A decision to treat PVCs in the inpatient convalescent phase after the third day should be based upon the
frequency and complexity of PVCs. Frequent PVCs (greater
than 6/min), bigeminy, trigeminy, or couplets or multifocal
PVCs should be treated with an oral antiarrhythmic drug,
assuming signs of reinfarction or recurrent ischemia are absent. In the presence of either of these situations, this
arrhythmia should be treated with intravenous lidocaine.

II. Atrial Arrhythmias

A. Sinus Tachycardia (Rate > 100 beats/min)

Although a benign arrhythmia, sinus tachycardia is actually
potentially serious in that it increases myocardial oxygen consumption and may, therefore, result in increased infarct size
or extension. If it is not the result of pain or emotional stress,
persistent sinus tachycardia usually indicates left ventricular
dysfunction and may be an early sign of congestive heart failure,
cardiogenic shock, or infarct extension. As such it may indicate
a poor prognosis. A treatable cause for the tachycardia should
be searched for and treated appropriately. If the sinus tachycardia is felt to be "inappropriate" and is not associated with
any signs of congestive heart failure, treatment with a beta-
blocker drug (if not otherwise contraindicated) is indicated to
decrease the heart rate. In the presence of congestive heart
failure, digitalization is sometimes effective for treatment of
tachycardia.

B. Sinus Bradycardia (Heart Rate < 60)

Sinus bradycardia is a common and usually transient arrhythmia
accompanying acute myocardial infarction, especially in the
presence of inferior wall myocardial infarction, due to increased vagal tone. When the sinus rate is over 40 beats/min,
no therapy is usually necessary unless symptoms or signs of
decreased perfusion are present such as hypotension, disturbed
sensorium, or congestive heart failure. Heart rates of less
than 40 are usually symptomatic and, like symptomatic sinus

bradycardia with rates over 40, should be treated. Initial
treatment consists of atropine, which can be given orally, sublingually, subcutaneously, intramuscularly, or intravenously.
For immediate response, the intravenous route is preferred.
The initial dose is 0.4 to 1.0 mg, depending on the degree of
bradycardia and/or hypotension. Since the duration of intravenous atropine is short, the dose may have to be repeated
frequently if the bradycardia returns. Since the side effects of
large doses of atropine usually prevent continued dosing, persistent symptomatic sinus bradycardia is best treated with the
insertion of a temporary transvenous pacemaker. Alternatively,
or as a temporary measure until a pacemaker can be inserted,
an intravenous infusion of isoproterenol can be started (0.5-2
μg/min), but this is often associated with unacceptable tachy-
arrhythmias and should only be used for short periods of
time and when absolutely necessary. Usually, significant sinus
bradycardia is a transient rhythm disturbance, lasting minutes
to hours, and does not require prolonged treatment.

   C.   Atrial and Junctional Premature Beats
        (PACs and PJCs)

Premature atrial beats and premature junctional beats, as well
as junctional tachycardia, are usually benign and do not have to
be treated, although very frequent premature atrial beats can
lead to the development of atrial fibrillation and in this instance
should be suppressed with quinidine or procainamide.

   D.   Atrial Fibrillation and Atrial Flutter

When either of these rhythms occur in the setting of acute myocardial infarction, the choice of treatment depends upon the
ventricular rate. Atrial fibrillation with a rapid rate (> 100)
presents the same increased oxygen demand on the heart that
sinus tachycardia does, with the additional problem of loss of
atrial contribution to cardiac output, both of which may be
particularly detrimental in patients with compromised left
ventricular function. If the patient is already on a drug which
decreases AV node conduction (digoxin or a beta-adrenergic
blocker or verapamil) or has an intrinsic AV node conduction
abnormality resulting in an acceptable ventricular rate, no
immediate treatment is usually necessary, as the rhythm is
in itself not dangerous and usually self-limited. If the rate
is over 100, however, immediate therapy is indicated. Depending upon the urgency of the situation (presence of chest
pain or other indication of ischemia, or cardiac decompensation),

either of two basic approaches can be taken: (1) for urgent situations, electrical synchronous cardioversion is the treatment of choice for either rapid atrial fibrillation or flutter; and (2) for less urgent situations, the rate should be controlled by a drug that blocks the AV node. Usually digoxin is preferred, although propranolol (or another beta-blocking drug) or verapamil can be used. Usually the intravenous route is preferred, although these drugs can be given orally if there is less urgency. Beta-blocking or calcium blocking drugs should be used with great caution in patients with evidence of congestive heart failure, hypotension, or intrinsic SA or AV node dysfunction.

Patients with acute myocardial infarction may be more sensitive to digoxin than other patients, and some caution must be used in dosing. For previously undigitalized patients, 0.50 mg is given intravenously, followed by 0.25 mg every 4-6 hours until the rate is slowed or normal sinus rhythm returns or a total of 1.5 mg is given. For propranolol, 1-8 mg is given intravenously at no more than 1 mg/min until the rate is slowed or hypotension occurs. For verapamil, 5-10 mg is given intravenously as a bolus. Repeat doses of propranolol or verapamil may be needed periodically depending upon the ventricular rate.

Atrial flutter presents a slightly different situation than fibrillation in that it is more difficult to slow the ventricular rate with digoxin and it is easier to convert electrically with low energy levels. With a healthy AV node, flutter usually conducts to the ventricle in a two to one fashion, so that the average ventricular rate is in the 140 to 160 range, which is not well tolerated by patients with acute myocardial infarction. Synchronous cardioversion (at a low energy level) is therefore the treatment of choice for this arrhythmia. If the conduction rate is four to one, with a resultant ventricular rate of 70-80, no treatment is usually necessary. Atrial flutter with variable conduction rates is similar to atrial fibrillation and should be approached the same way. Once the ventricular rate is controlled with either of these rhythms, if spontaneous conversion to normal sinus rhythm does not occur, conversion can be done electively at a later time, using pharmacologic means (usually quinidine or procainamide) or electrical cardioversion.

Table 8-1 summarizes the approach to atrial and ventricular arrhythmias in the setting of acute myocardial infarction.

CONDUCTION DEFECTS

First Degree Heart Block (Prolonged P-R Interval)

First degree heart block is a benign A-V conduction defect that is often seen in acute inferior wall myocardial infarction. It

Table 8-1. Management of Arrhythmias in Acute MI

Arrhythmia	Modifying Factors	Initial Treatment	Subsequent Treatment
Ventricular Fibrillation		**Defibrillation – 400 W. S.**	Lidocaine bolus and drip
Ventricular Tachycardia	Rate ≥ 150 or signs of cardiac decompensation	Defibrillation – 400 W. S.	Lidocaine bolus and drip
	Rate ≤ 140 and no signs of cardiac decompensation	Lidocaine bolus (100 mg)	Lidocaine drip, (2-4 mg/min)
Accelerated idioventricular		Eliminate any contributing cause	
PVCs		Lidocaine bolus (50-100 mg)	Lidocaine drip
PACs	Infrequent	No treatment necessary	
	Frequent (≥ 10 minuute)	Quinidine 200-300 mg q 6 h or Procainamide 250-500 mg q 4 h	Same

Sinus Bradycardia	Rate > 45 and asymptomatic	No treatment necessary
	Rate < 45 or symptomatic	Atropine 0.4-1.0 mg I.V. or Isoproterenol 1-4 μg/min	Temporary transvenous pacemaker if necessary
Sinus Tachycardia	Rate < 120 and asymptomatic	Sedation, if necessary	Propranolol if persistent
	Rate > 120 or symptomatic	Treat specific cause	Propranolol or digoxin
Atrial Fibrillation	VR* < 100 and asymptomatic	Digoxin (P.O. or I.V.)	Digoxin
	VR > 100 or symptomatic	Digoxin (I.V.)	Quinidine or
	VR > 140	Cardioversion	Procainamide
Atrial Flutter	VR < 90 (4:1 or 3:1 block)	No treatment necessary	Digoxin and Quinidine or Cardio-version
	VR > 90 (2:1 or 3:1 block)	Cardioversion	Quinidine

*VR = Ventricular Rate

does not require therapy but may indicate subsequent second degree AV block, which often does require treatment. Drugs
which may further prolong AV conduction should be used with
caution or discontinued (digoxin, beta-blocking drugs, or verapamil or diltiazem).

Second Degree AV Block

Second degree AV block is a conduction defect that is also common in acute inferior wall myocardial infarction and is usually
transient. It can appear as a Wenckebach phenomenon (Mobitz
type-1 block) or as a fixed type of block (2:1, 3:1, etc.). As in
sinus bradycardia, treatment is dependent upon the ventricular
rate and clinical situation. If the rate is acceptable and there
are no apparent adverse physical consequences, no treatment is
usually necessary. If the rate is excessively low ($<$ 45 beats/
min), atropine is usually given and often restores 1:1 conduction. If this condition is persistent and symptomatic, a temporary pacemaker is indicated.

Third Degree AV Block

Third degree AV block can be due to transient AV node dysfunction, as is the case in first degree and second degree AV
block (usually in the setting of acute inferior wall myocardial
infarction), or can be due to infranodal dysfunction resulting
from infarction of the bundle branches (usually seen in large
anteroseptal infarctions), in which case it is often permanent.
In AV nodal dysfunction, there is usually an adequate junctional
escape rate, and this can be managed with atropine, or with a
temporary pacemaker if necessary. With infranodal dysfunction,
there is usually an inadequate ventricular escape rate and coexisting left ventricular dysfunction. This type of block is
unresponsive to atropine and requires temporary pacing (and
usually subsequent implantation of a permanent pacemaker),
although the almost uniform severe left ventricular dysfunction
seen in this setting due to massive infarction usually leads to a
poor prognosis despite correction of the heart block.

Bundle Branch (Fascicular) Blocks

The sudden appearance of a bundle branch block (left or right)
with or without axis deviation in a setting of acute anteroseptal
myocardial infarction has a somewhat similar, if less ominous,
significance as the appearance of complete heart block. That is,
buncle branch block is due to infarction in the septum which may

suddenly progress to complete heart block with extension of the infarction. The indication for prophylactic insertion of a temporary (if not permanent) pacemaker is still controversial in this setting. The appearance of trifascicular block (right bundle branch with left or right axis deviation and first degree A-V block, or left bundle branch block with first degree A-V block, or alternating right and left bundle branch block) should always be treated with insertion of a temporary pacemaker. The bifascicular block pattern combinations of right bundle branch block with left anterior hemiblock or left posterior hemiblock or first degree A-V block also carries a significant risk of subsequent third degree heart block and should be treated with temporary pacemaker insertion. Even isolated, new complete right bundle or left bundle branch blocks frequently proceed to complete heart block in the setting of anterior myocardial infarction and should be managed with a temporary prophylactic pacemaker (Table 8-2).

HYPERTENSION

Systolic hypertension often accompanies the early stages of acute myocardial infarction, and both systolic and diastolic hypertension tend to be accentuated in previously hypertensive patients, even in those in whom the hypertension has been under good control with medical treatment. This occurs as a result of increased circulating catecholamines and sympathetic discharge associated with the stress of acute myocardial infarction and is usually self-limited. Since even transient severe hypertension results in increased myocardial oxygen demand and may increase the possibility of infarct extension and of myocardial rupture, immediate treatment of severe hypertension is mandatory. The choice of treatment depends upon the degree of blood pressure elevation as well as upon the overall clinical situation. Very often the treatment of acute elevation of blood pressure due to a stress reaction consists merely of reducing the stress and pain with analgesics and tranquilizers. If this is only partially successful, a single dose of a nitrate or a diuretic may provide the additional necessary reduction of blood pressure. If the patient is not in congestive heart failure, an alternate choice of therapy is a beta-blocking drug, which is particularly useful if the patient has tachycardia in addition. Propranolol may be given intravenously in small increments if necessary, otherwise any of the beta-blockers can be given orally. Alternatively, if the hypertension is mild to moderate and the patient is clinically stable, any of the standard antihypertensive medications which do not cause a reflex tachycardia can be used.

Table 8-2. Management of Conduction Abnormalities in Acute MI

Abnormality	Modifying Factors	Initial Treatment	Subsequent Treatment
1 A-V Block		No treatment necessary	
2 A-V Block	Mobitz-1, Inferior MI, asymptomatic	Discontinue any contributing drugs	Usually self-limited
	VR < 45 or symptomatic	Atropine 0.4-1 mg I.V.	Temporary pacemaker if necessary
3 A-V Block	Mobitz-2, Anterior MI	Temporary pacemaker	Permanent pacemaker
	Inferior MI, VR > 45, asymptomatic	Careful observation	Usually self-limited
	Inferior MI, VR < 45 or symptomatic	Atropine 0.4-1.0 mg I.V.	Temporary pacemaker if persistent

Bundle Branch Blocks	Anterior MI	Temporary pacemaker	Permanent pacemaker
	Isolated LBBB or RBBB	Careful observation	Permanent pacemaker if 2° or 3° AV block develops
	Bifascicular block (New)	Temporary pacemaker	Observation
	Trifascicular block (New)	Temporary pacemaker	Permanent pacemaker

In other instances, where the hypertension is severe and
sustained or when it is markedly fluctuating, or the patient is
having considerable pain or is otherwise unstable, intravenous
infusion of a rapidly acting antihypertensive medication is the
treatment of choice, using either nitroprusside or nitroglycerin.
The latter is a good choice if preload reduction is also desired
for control of chest pain or congestive heart failure. The dose
of either of these drugs is adjusted according to response, with
the dose range of nitroprusside being 20-200 μg/min and
nitroglycerin from 5-100 or more μg/min. The blood pressure
needs to be monitored continuously with either intravenous infusion, using either direct intraarterial blood pressure monitoring, or an automatic blood pressure cuff device. Hypotension
needs to be avoided as much as severe hypertension to avoid
hypoperfusion of the coronary arteries. In general, blood pressure should be maintained at "normal" levels (120-140 systolic
and 60-80 mm diastolic) if at all possible. Patients should be
switched to oral medications as soon as stabilized, and intravenous infusions should gradually be reduced and discontinued.

HYPOTENSION AND SHOCK

Hypotension generally refers to a systolic blood pressure of less
than 90-100 or a fall in systolic blood pressure to 30 mm below
the patient's usual blood pressure. Hypotension is not synony-
mous with shock, since shock includes, in addition to hypotension, signs of inadequate arterial perfusion: change in mental
status, decrease in urine output, and cool and clammy skin.
Cardiogenic shock (shock resultant from inadequate cardiac
output due to massive myocardial infarction) is associated with
a very high mortality, whereas hypotension without shock is
usually reversible. Hypotension in acute myocardial infarction
may be due to hypovolemia (especially if the patient has been
nauseated and vomiting), to reflex vasodilatation, to low cardiac
output, or to a combination of these factors. If hypovolemia
seems likely on the basis of history and physical examination,
an empiric trial of volume infusion can be initiated, giving
normal saline, low molecular weight dextran, or 5% albumin
in boluses of 100 ml until blood pressure is normalized or a
maximum of 500 ml has been given. If reflex hypotension
seems likely on the basis of accompanying bradycardia and other
signs of increased vagal tone, this should be corrected with
intravenous atropine (0.4 - 1 mg). If low cardiac output seems
likely or the cause is unclear, a thermister-tipped, flow-
directed pulmonary artery catheter (Swan-Ganz) should be inserted if at all possible in order to determine the left ventricular

HEMODYNAMIC EVALUATION AND TREATMENT OF HYPOTENSION

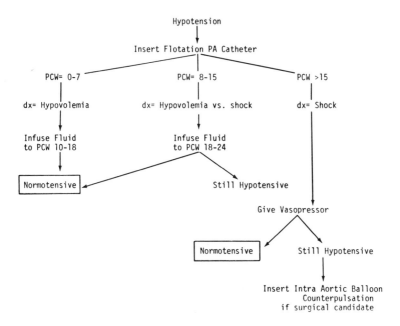

Figure 8-10.   Evaluation and management of hypotension in acute myocardial infarction.

filling pressure (pulmonary capillary wedge pressure) and cardiac output. A normal wedge pressure is between 8 and 12 mmHg, while in hypovolemic states, the wedge pressure is under 8 mmHg, and in congestive states, the wedge pressure is over 15 mmHg. The normal cardiac index (cardiac output divided by body surface area) is between 2.5 and 3.5 $L/min/M^2$. In a hypotensive patient with a low wedge pressure and low cardiac output, a volume expander should be infused until the wedge pressure and blood pressure are within normal range. If the wedge pressure is normal and the cardiac output and blood pressure are low, a volume infusion may still be effective, since a higher than normal filling pressure (15-18 mmHg) may be necessary in a failing heart. Volume should not be infused beyond a wedge pressure of 18 mmHg, however, in order to avoid putting the patient into congestive heart failure. If the wedge pressure is high and the cardiac output and blood pressure are low, the patient is in cardiogenic shock and needs to be treated with a vasopressor and inotropic drugs or balloon counterpulsation (Figure 8-10).

Table 8-3.   Comparative Effects of Vasopressor Drugs

Drug	Blood Pressure	Heart Rate	Contractility	Renal Blood Flow	Arrhythmias
Norepine-phrine	++++	++	++	---	++
Dopamine	++*	++	+++	+++	+++
Dobutamine	++**	+	+++	+	+

+ = increase; - = decrease
  *Due to increased cardiac output at lower doses and to vaso-
   constriction at higher doses.
**Increase in blood pressure due entirely to increased cardiac
   output.

Vasopressors and Inotropic Drugs (Table 8-3)

The most commonly employed vasopressors are the catecholamines: norepinephrine, dopamine, and dobutamine.

1. Norepinephrine

Norepinephrine is an inotropic agent with both alpha and beta-
adrenergic stimulating effects when given in usual doses. This
is usually the drug of choice for initial therapy of severe hypotension (blood pressure less than 70) and is usually given in a
concentration of 4 μg/ml and titrated according to response,
starting with 4 μg/min and increasing to a maximum dose of
32 μg/min. Like all beta-adrenergic stimulants, it has the
undesirable side effects of increased heart rate and irritability
as well as the desired effect of increased cardiac contractility.

2. Dopamine

This catecholamine also has alpha and beta effects, with the
beta effect predominating at lower doses and the alpha at higher
doses. In addition, in contrast to norepinephrine, it produces
renal and mesenteric vasodilatation at low to moderate doses.
It is a very useful drug in patients with cardiogenic shock with
systolic blood pressures between 70 and 90 mmHg. The usual

starting dose is 0.2 mg/min, with the usual range varying from this to 4 mg/min according to patient response. As with norepinephrine, tachycardia and cardiac arrhythmias are often seen as side effects.

   3. Dobutamine

Dobutamine is a synthetic catecholamine producing an increase in contractility without significant effects on vascular tone or heart rate. It is therefore most useful in mild to moderate hypotension (systolic blood pressure 70-90) in which improvement of contractility alone is sufficient to reverse the shock picture. The starting dose is 0.2 mg/min, with the usual range being from 0.2-1 mg/min.

Use of Intraaortic Balloon Counterpulsation (IABCP)

This technique, which has been in use for a number of years, is a very useful temporary method of supporting a failing heart and reversing cardiogenic shock. The device consists of an inflatable balloon on an intravascular catheter which is automatically inflated with helium during diastole and deflated during systole by means of an external synchronized pump. This results in an "unloading" of the ventricle during ventricular systole and augmentation of coronary and systemic perfusion during diastole. The balloon is inserted into the femoral artery by surgical cutdown or by percutaneous technique and is advanced and positioned in the thoracic aorta. Insertion of the balloon catheter should generally be reserved for situations which are potentially reversible, such as cardiogenic shock due to surgically repairable lesions (ruptured chordae, ruptured interventricular septum, or ruptured free wall), or severe ischemia in the setting of acute myocardial infarction, or cardiogenic shock in early acute myocardial infarction which might still be reversible with coronary bypass surgery. Although some patients in cardiogenic shock due to massive and irreversible myocardial infarction can be maintained for a considerable time with this technique, little is to be gained by this approach if the heart cannot function adequately once the pump is discontinued.

CONGESTIVE HEART FAILURE
AND PULMONARY EDEMA

Severe congestive heart failure and pulmonary edema are common consequences of acute myocardial infarction, especially when the infarction is large or is in the setting of compromised left ventricular function from previous infarction or from hypertension or mechanical complications (mitral regurgitation or ventricular septal rupture). Acute pulmonary edema is the most severe form of congestive heart failure and must be treated quickly and aggressively to avoid irreversible complications. It is characterized by severe dyspnea and tachycardia, cyanosis, diaphoresis, wheezing, distended neck veins, extensive rales, and usually an S3 gallop. Treatment consists of administration of oxygen by mask (5 l/min), administration of morphine sulphate (2-10 mg titrated intravenously), furosemide (40 mg intravenously), and, if necessary, rotating tourniquets.

Lesser degrees of congestive heart failure manifested by mild to moderate dyspnea, neck-vein distension, rales covering less than half of the lower lung fields, and with or without an S3 gallop, should also be treated, but without the same urgency and intensity as acute pulmonary edema. The key to treatment is diuresis, which can be accomplished with intravenous or oral diuretics (usually using furosemide, although other diuretics can be used). Digitalis is usually not very helpful in the initial treatment of acute heart failure in the setting of acute myocardial infarction. Nitrates are also helpful as ancillary treatment in the treatment of congestive heart failure, by further reducing preload, and can be given orally, sublingually, topically, or intravenously.

In patients with refractory heart failure, especially in the setting of elevated blood pressure, the use of afterload (blood pressure) reducing agents may be indicated. In this group of patients, a flow-directed pulmonary artery (Swan-Ganz) catheter should be inserted to monitor pulmonary capillary wedge pressure and cardiac output, and arterial pressure should be monitored by an arterial catheter or automatic blood pressure cuff. In all cases of left-sided heart failure, the wedge pressure is abnormally elevated, usually in the range of 20-30 mmHg. The cardiac output is usually but not necessarily reduced. There is usually elevation of the systemic vascular resistance (calculated by the formula SVR = mean arterial blood pressure minus mean right atrial pressure, divided by cardiac output, and multiplied by 80, with normal values being in the range of 800-1200 dynes/sec/cm^5). Afterload reduction therapy is indicated if systemic vascular resistance is abnormally high and the cardiac output is low. Effective treatment should reverse these derangements with a decrease in SVR and increase in cardiac output. Wedge pressure may also decrease as a result of improved left ventricular function.

There are several antihypertensive drugs in common use as afterload reduction agents in acute myocardial infarction:

intravenous nitroglycerin, sodium nitroprusside (Nipride), hydralazine (Apresoline), and prazosin (Minipress). (Captopril [Capoten] is also an effective drug for reduction of afterload and preload but should be used cautiously in the setting of acute myocardial infarction.) Sodium nitroprusside also results in a fall of left ventricular filling pressure due to venous dilatation and pooling in additional to arterial dilatation. This drug is given intravenously (20-200 μg/min) as a continuous infusion and allows fine control of SVR, as it has a rapid onset and offset and can be titrated according to response.

Hydralazine can also be given both parenterally (intravenously or intramuscularly) and orally and results in arterial dilatation without significant venous dilatation and is often combined with nitrates or diuretics to reduce filling pressure in addition to increasing cardiac output. In the setting of severe heart failure in acute infarction with increased SVR and decreased cardiac output, this drug may be given intravenously if pulmonary artery and arterial monitoring lines are in place. A test dose of 10 mg is given over a 20-30-minute period intravenously by infusion, and if tolerated, the dose is increased to 25-100 mg intravenously every 6 hours according to response. If successful, the patient then can be switched to oral hydralazine in similar dosages. Alternatively, if the situation is less urgent, the patient can be started on oral hydralazine initially. Alternatively, prazosin (Minipress) can be given, which provides both arterial and venous dilatation, similar to nitroprusside. This drug is given orally only with the dose being determined empirically, usually in the range of 1-5 mg every 8-12 hours. With all of these agents, SVR and cardiac output are monitored, with the goal of maximization of cardiac output but avoidance of hypotension.

Congestive Heart Failure due to Right Ventricular Infarction

Infarction of the right ventricle often accompanies inferior wall myocardial infarction. Although this is usually of no clinical significance, severe right ventricular infarction can result in a picture of severe right-sided congestive heart failure, often with systemic hypotension as well. This syndrome is clinically diagnosed by severe jugular venous distension as a result of elevated right atrial pressure. Hemodynamic measurements, if done, reveal elevated right atrial and right ventricular diastolic pressures disproportionate to elevations in pulmonary artery and pulmonary wedge pressures. If hypotension is present, volume expanders should be infused despite the high right-sided pressures until the hypotension is corrected or the wedge pressure is in the 15-20 mm range.

OTHER COMPLICATIONS OF
ACUTE MYOCARDIAL INFARCTION

The sudden appearance of severe congestive heart failure or cardiogenic shock with or without accompanying new chest pain in the course of acute infarction should arouse suspicion of one of the following complications: (1) recurrent (extension of) infarction, (2) rupture of chordae tendinae or the tip of a papillary muscle, with subsequent severe mitral regurgitation, (3) rupture of the ventricular septum with resultant left to right shunt, or (4) free wall myocardial rupture. The initial steps toward differential diagnosis consist of careful reexamination of the patient and repeating the electrocardiogram. In the case of recurrent myocardial infarction, there are no specific physical findings, but the electrocardiogram is usually diagnostic, showing new ST segment elevations (or in the case of subendo-cardial infarction, ST segment depressions). In the case of rupture of the chordae tendinae, papillary muscle, or ventricu-lar septum, the key to diagnosis is the sudden appearance of a new and loud holosystolic murmur at the apex or left sternal border. The differentiation of these two complications is best made by the insertion of a Swan-Ganz catheter: in mitral regurgitation the key to diagnosis is the presence of large v waves in the wedge pressure tracing, whereas in ventricular septal rupture, the key finding is a left to right shunt at the ventricular level detected by an abnormally high right ventric-ular oxygen saturation compared to the right atrium. In the case of free wall myocardial rupture, there is usually sudden cardiovascular collapse despite normal rhythm and absence of a new murmur or evidence of extension of the myocardial infarction on the electrocardiogram. In this setting, this diagnosis should always be considered, and an emergency pericardiocentesis should be attempted to relieve the associated cardiac tamponade. Although the prognosis of this complica-tion is very poor, there have been reports of patients being salvaged by emergency surgery (surgical repair of the rupture). In the case of ventricular septal rupture or severe mitral regurgitation, surgery is also indicated with temporary medical support by treatment of congestive heart failure with afterload reduction or treatment of shock with a vasopressor. Infarct extension resulting in severe congestive heart failure or shock should be treated with medical support as discussed earlier.

Pericarditis

Acute pericarditis is a common manifestation of transmural
acute infarction and is seen within the first 4 days. It may be
mild and asymptomatic or may be more severe with chest pain,
fever, and atrial arrhythmias. Physical examination discloses
a pericardial friction rub, and the electrocardiogram often
shows diffuse ST segment elevations. Most cases do not require treatment, but symptomatic cases can be treated with
aspirin or indomethacin.

Dressler's syndrome (postmyocardial infarction syndrome)
also consists of pericarditis which usually occurs later than
the acute pericarditis of myocardial infarction (typically in the
second or third week after the infarction) and is usually symptomatic, with pleural-pericardial chest pain, fever, and often
pleural effusions (usually left sided) and/or pulmonary infil-
trates. Although uncommon, pericardial tamponade can occur.
An elevation in white blood cell count and sedimentation rate is
typical, and echocardiography confirms the presence of
pericardial fluid. Treatment is indicated, with aspirin or
indomethacin, and if the patient is unresponsive to either of
these, treatment with a corticosteroid is indicated (40-60 mg
of prednisone/day for 1 week, with gradual tapering there-
after). This condition is often confused with acute pulmonary
embolization, which may have a similar clinical presentation
except for the pericardial rub and pericardial effusion, which
are not usual features of acute pulmonary embolus. A ventila-
tion-perfusion lung scan should be obtained to differentiate
these two conditions. Dressler's syndrome tends to be recurrent over a period of months or even years and may need
several courses of treatment with antiinflammatory drugs.

Arterial and Venous Thromboembolism

Deep venous thrombosis in the lower extremities is common
during acute myocardial infarction, particularly in patients
with congestive heart failure or those subjected to prolonged
bed rest. Subsequent pulmonary emboli is an uncommon but
potentially serious complication. The incidence of these complications can be decreased by early mobilization of the uncomplicated patient and by prophylactic low-dose heparin
administration (5,000-7,500 units subcutaneously every 12
hours) in patients with congestive heart failure, obesity,
chronic venous disease, or in need of prolonged bed rest.

Left ventricular mural thrombus formation at the site of
infarction is also common but rarely results in arterial embolization. It is not known whether prophylactic minidose or

higher dose heparin decreases the incidence of mural thrombus formation and embolization. If embolization does occur, therapeutic heparinization is instituted immediately and maintained from 7-10 days, after which oral anticoagulation with warfarin (Coumadin) is begun.

Recurrent Chest Pain

Although normally the acute pain associated with myocardial infarction subsides after the first day, pain may recur during the subsequent course of convalescence and can be due to a variety of causes, including recurrent infarction, episodes of ischemia, pericarditis, and pulmonary emboli. The diagnosis and treatment of the latter two conditions has already been commented upon. The differentiation of recurrent infarction from ischemic episodes is based upon the electrocardiographic and enzymatic criteria discussed earlier. The treatment of recurrent infarction is the same as for initial infarction. Recurrent ischemia is characterized by chest pain of variable duration, usually accompanied by ST segment or T wave changes, and is usually at least partially reversible by nitroglycerin. When recurrent ischemia is diagnosed following acute myocardial infarction, it needs to be treated aggressively to prevent infarct extension. Contributing factors such as hypertension, heart failure, tachycardia, and anemia should be treated if present to decrease the degree of ischemia. Treatment with nitrates, beta-blockers, and calcium blockers follows the same guidelines outlined in Chapter 7, and arteriography may need to be done despite recent infarction if pain cannot be readily controlled with medication and if reinfarction seems likely, in order to evaluate the possible need and feasibility for coronary bypass surgery.

MANAGEMENT OF THE EARLY CONVALESCENT PHASE OF ACUTE MYOCARDIAL INFARCTION — GENERAL PRINCIPLES

Once the patient has survived the first 2 to 3 days of an uncomplicated myocardial infarction or has recovered from the complications of a complicated infarction, he is considered to be in the convalescent phase. Although the patient usually does not need the degree of professional attention required in the first few days of hospitalization, a coordinated and comprehensive approach to convalescence is a necessary prerequisite to successful management and preparation for discharge. The following categories need to be considered: diet, activity, arrhythmia detection, medication, and psychological support.

DIET

As in the initial diet, the diet should be on an individual basis. In the absence of congestive heart failure or hypertension, there is no need to restrict sodium, but the patient should in general be encouraged to reduce his dietary intake of sodium, particularly in the presence of borderline hypertension or heart failure. Similarly, although there is no need to acutely lower cholesterol and fat intake, the in-hospital rehabilitation phase may be a good opportunity to reeducate patients on a prudent diet. As in the acute phase, the quantity of food intake should be appropriate for metabolic needs, and the activity level and the total intake should be spread out into three or four balanced meals.

ACTIVITY

Activity levels need to be individually determined for each patient on a daily basis. An uncomplicated patient can be permitted to sit in a chair on the third or fourth hospital day, while a more complicated patient might be at complete bed rest for 5 to 7 days. If the patient's blood pressure and heart-rate response to leg dangling in bed on the second or third hospital day are normal and he otherwise tolerates this well, he can be permitted to sit in a chair for meals, with bed rest at other times. During the first few days, a bedside commode is preferable to bathroom use, to limit energy expenditure, but if the patient is doing well, he may be permitted to use the bathroom for bowel movements provided it is only a few steps from the bed and rhythm monitoring can be done. Washing and bathing should still be done in bed. The patient should not shave himself during the first few days, but this can be done for him. During the first week, simple physical conditioning exercises should be taught to the patient and performed in bed or in a chair several times per week.

After the first week, the speed of progression of activities also depends upon the condition of the patient. Those patients who remain asymptomatic, especially if they were fairly active prior to the infarction, can be progressed quickly so that they are up "ad lib" in the room by the fourth or fifth hospital day, with full bathroom privileges, and are ambulating freely by the seventh to tenth day and ready for discharge at this time. Other patients may take 3 or more weeks to achieve the same level.

On the average, an uncomplicated or minimally complicated patient can be discharged by the tenth hospital day. Table 8-4 gives examples of activity levels and physical therapy levels used during convalescence from acute myocardial infarction.

Should the patient experience a setback during the hospitalization such as recurrence of chest pain or another complication, the activity level may need to be reduced temporarily or maintained at a certain level for a longer than usual time until the patient is again recuperating smoothly.

TREATMENT OF ARRHYTHMIAS

As discussed previously, the likelihood of serious arrhythmias is greatest in the first 2 to 3 days after an acute infarction. However, later occurrences of arrhythmias are not uncommon, especially premature ventricular beats. Late hospital ventricular fibrillation, however, is quite uncommon, even in the presence of frequent premature beats. Therefore, the need for continued monitoring in patients free of arrhythmias after the first few days depends to an extent on the approach to treatment of asymptomatic premature beats in thos population. If feasible, all postmyocardial infarction patients could be maintained on cardiac monitors throughout their hospital course (with the use of telemetry) in order to detect late arrhythmias and to initiate and evaluate response to antiarrhythmic therapy. This is not feasible in most hospitals, however, and an alternate approach would be to monitor uncomplicated patients only for the first 3 to 5 days and to do a predischarge Holter monitor or function stress test (see below) in order to detect prognostically significant arrhythmias. The treatment of these late arrhythmias is still controversial and was discussed earlier.

PSYCHOLOGICAL SUPPORT

This is one area that is often ignored by physicians or left to other hospital personnel, but it is a very important component of the successful rehabilitation of the patient. Most patients experience some sort of psychological stress during their hospitalization. Initial shock, anxiety, or disbelief may become depression or despair. Frequent reassurance is often necessary to convince the patient that he will most likely not be permanently incapacitated by his infarction, and that after a period of convalescence, in most cases, he can return to work and to a completely normal life-style. Continued encouragement by the physician, nurses, and other hospital personnel can be very useful for the patient and the family as

Table 8-4. Activity Levels in Acute MI

Level	Day	METS*	Activities
1	1	1	Complete bed rest; bed bath by nurse.
2	1-2	1.5	Bedside commode; may feed self.
3	2-3	1.5-2	Dangle legs on side of bed b.i.d.; may wash hands and face in bed.
4	3-4	2	Sit in chair b.i.d. with meals; partial bath in bed.
5	4-5	2.5	Sit in chair t.i.d. - q.i.d.; bathroom privileges for B.M.
6	5-6	2.5-3	Walk in room; full B.R.P.
7	6-7	3	Walk in hall up to 5 minutes b.i.d. - t.i.d.; bath in tub.
8	7-10	3-3.5	Walk in hall up to 10 minutes b.i.d. - t.i.d.; shower on seat.
9	10-14	3.5-4	Walk in hall as desired; shower.
10	10-14	4	Low level exercise test.

*1 MET = Energy expenditure at rest
Compiled from Cardiac Rehabilitation Programs in use at
Cedars-Sinai, U.C.L.A., Brotman, and Midway Medical
Centers, Los Angeles, CA

well. Although tranquilizing drugs may be necessary and desirable in the first few days of hospitalization, most patients
do not require continued use of these agents beyond this.

PREDISCHARGE EXERCISE STRESS TESTING

Over the past few years, the safety and prognostic value of predischarge (or early postdischarge) exercise stress testing has
been established for patients recovering from acute myocardial

infarction. Known as a low-level or function exercise test, several protocols are in common use, using reduced levels of exercise compared to diagnostic submaximal or maximal stress tests. In contrast to the target heart rate of 85-90% of maximum predicted heart rate used for submaximal exercise testing, the function test uses a maximum of 70-75% of age-predicted maximal heart rate or uses symptom limitation if this heart rate is not achieved. In one protocol, the speed of the treadmill is kept constant at 2 miles/hr, and the grade is increased every 2 or 3 minutes by 3.5% increments. This test is done in patients who are fully ambulatory and ready for discharge and are uncomplicated (no congestive heart failure or significant arrhythmia or conduction defects). Patients with poor exercise tolerance or with a positive test (ST segment depression or elevation with or without chest pain) tend to have multivessel disease, poor left ventricular function, and a five to ten times worse prognosis than patients with longer exercise tolerance or negative tests, and this differentiation may be useful in deciding which patients to consider for early angiography and consideration of coronary bypass surgery. There is also some evidence that patients with frequent premature ventricular beats in exercise testing have a worse 1-year prognosis than patients without this finding, and this may be helpful in deciding which patients to put on antiarrhythmic therapy after infarction. In addition, function testing is helpful in individualizing discharge exercise rehabilitation planning (see Chapter 9).

PREDISCHARGE COUNSELING

Instructions on diet, activity, and medications vary with the individual patient but follow general guidelines.

DIET

The discharge diet should generally be the same as during the latter period of hospitalization. Uncomplicated patients without any evidence of heart failure or hypertension can be on a regular salt diet, although they should be encouraged to minimize their salt intake in general. The issue of low-fat and low-cholesterol diet is considered in Chapter 11. Although the number of calories should be appropriate to the activity level, patients should not go on a severe low-calorie diet for weight reduction during the recuperative phase of acute infarction.

ACTIVITY

Because of the initial excitement and stress of discharge and being at home for the first time in 1 or more weeks, patients should be cautioned to minimize their activities during the first few days at home, but should be encouraged to be up and around the house. If a patient lives in a two-story house, he should be advised to minimize his daily trips up and down the stairs. After the first few days, he can start to venture outdoors for short walks, starting with one block each way once or twice a day at a leisurely pace, and progressing in distance and pace according to how well the exercise is tolerated. By the end of the second week at home, most patients can walk one-quarter to one-half mile in each direction without difficulty. Short automobile rides are permissible after the first few days at home, but driving is not advised for at least 4 weeks of recuperation. Sexual activity is permissible after 3 to 6 weeks of recuperation (when a heart rate of 120 is tolerated without symptoms). The patients should ordinarily be seen in follow-up in the physician's office in 10-14 days after discharge.

MEDICATION

Ordinarily, medications taken in the hospital at the time of discharge should be continued after discharge, including medications to prevent reinfarction (discussed above). Indications for continued use of various medications that were started in the hospital need to be reviewed periodically in the physician's office.

RETURN TO WORK

The time taken to return to employment obviously depends upon the type of employment as well as the condition of the patient and his rate of progress. On the average, patients return to work about 3 months from the time of their acute infarction, but this time varies from 6 weeks to 6 months in individual cases. In general, it is advisable to do a submaximal stress test prior to returning to any work which requires significant physical exertion in order to ascertain whether there is any residual evidence of exercise-induced ischemia or arrhythmias.

PROGNOSIS AFTER MYOCARDIAL INFARCTION

Prognosis after myocardial infarction can be divided into early (prehospital and hospital) and late (postdischarge) categories.

The incidence of sudden (instantaneous) death from acute
coronary thrombosis before enough time has elapsed for myocardial infarction to occur is unknown but may be as high as
50%. Once a patient has survived long enough to reach the
hospital, the overall mortality during hospitalization is approximately 15%, with most of the deaths due to severe left ventricular dysfunction (heart failure and/or shock) and refractory
arrhythmias. Depending upon a number of clinical factors,
patients can be divided into a very low-risk group, with an in-
hospital mortality of less than 5%, an intermediate-risk group,
and a high-risk group, with a mortality of approximately 80%.
In general, this categorization can be determined within the
first few days admission, allowing a less aggressive approach
and a shorter hospital stay for the very low-risk group. Major
factors which determine the risk are listed below:

	Low Risk	Intermediate Risk	High Risk
Age	< 50	50-69	≥ 70
Location of MI	Nontransmural	Inferior	Anterior
Systolic BP	> 100	85-100	< 85
Heart Size	Normal	Borderline	Enlarged
Heart Failure	None	Mild-Moderate	Severe
LV Ejection Fraction	> 50%	40-50%	< 40%
Hemodynamics	Normal PCW + CI	Normal PCW + Low CI	High PCW + Low CI
Size of MI (Peak CK)	Small	Moderate	Large

Having survived the hospitalization phase of acute myocardial infarction, there is still a significant postdischarge
mortality, with an average 1-year mortality of 10% (most of
which occurs in the first 6 months), with an additional 5%
mortality in the second year, and a 3-4% mortality each subsequent year. Since there may be medical and surgical modalities
to decrease this mortality, it is important to recognize which
patients are in the high-risk groups. As is the case for acute
hospital-phase mortality, a number of clinical and other factors
have been recognized which help to differentiate these groups.
All of the factors listed above are also important determinants
of late prognosis, although patients with nontransmural (subendocardial) infarction who survive hospitalization tend to have
a higher late mortality than patients with transmural infarction, due to recurrent infarction and sudden death.

In addition to the above factors, a number of other factors
have been identified which contribute to late risk mortality.

These include postinfarction angina, significant late hospital arrhythmias, history of prior myocardial infarction, angina pectoris, stroke, diabetes mellitus, hypertension, elevated BUN, in-hospital development of heart failure, persistent sinus tachycardia, development of bundle branch block or complete heart block (in anterior MIs), and evidence of ischemia or significant arrhythmias on low-level exercise testing. In addition, evidence of significant ischemia (especially in an area remote from the acute infarction) on thallium stress testing also appears to be an indicator of poor prognosis.

The decision to proceed with further workup (coronary arteriography) and possible coronary artery bypass surgery or coronary angioplasty in these high-risk patients is discussed in Chapter 10.

REFERENCES

GENERAL

Alpert, J. S. and Braunwald, E.: Pathological and clinical manifestations of acute myocardial infarction, in Braunwald, E. (Ed.), "Heart Disease," W. B. Saunders, Philadelphia, 1980, pp. 1309-1359.

Genton, E. and Turpie, A. G. G.: Anticoagulant therapy following acute myocardial infarction. Mod Conc Cardiovasc Dis 52, 1983, pp. 45-51.

Hurst, J. W., King, S. B. III, Walter, P. F., Friesinger, G. C., and Edwards, J. E.: Atherosclerotic coronary heart disease: angina pectoris, myocardial infarction and other manifestations of myocardial ischemia, in Hurst, J. W. (Ed.), "The Heart," McGraw-Hill, New York, 1982, pp. 1010-1149.

Karliner, J. S. and Gregoratus, G. (Eds.): "Coronary Care," Churchill Livingstone, New York, 1981, pp. 127-558.

Norris, R. E.: "Myocardial Infarction. Its Presentation, Pathogenesis and Treatment," Churchill Livingstone, Edinburgh, 1982, p. 322.

Pryor, D. B., Hindman, M. C., Wagner, G. S., Califf, R. M., Rhoads, M. K., and Rosati, R. A.: Early discharge after myocardial infarction. Ann Intern Med 99, 1983, pp. 528-538.

Rackley, C. E. , Russell, R. O. Jr. , Mantle, J. A. , Rogers, W. J. , and Papapietro, S. E. : Modern approach to myocardial infarction: Determination of prognosis and therapy. Am Heart J 101, 1981, pp. 75-85.

Sleight, P. and Sobel, B. (Eds.): "The Pathophysiology and Management of Heart Disease, 2. Myocardial infarction." Medi-Cine, London, 1981.

Sobel, B. E. and Braunwald, E. : The management of acute myocardial infarction, in Braunwald, E. (Ed.), "Heart Disease," W. B. Saunders, Philadelphia, 1980, pp. 1353-1386.

Wenger, N. K. : Uncomplicated acute myocardial infarction: long term management. Ann Intern Med 52, 1983, pp. 658-660.

LIMITATION OF INFARCT SIZE
(STREPTOKINASE AND OTHER METHODS)

Anderson, J. L. , Marshall, H. W. , Bray, B. E. , Lutz, J. R. , Frederick, P. R. , Yanowitz, F. G. , Datz, F. L. , Klausner, S. C. , and Hagen, A. D. : A randomized trial of intracoronary streptokinase in the treatment of acute myocardial infarction. N Engl J Med 308, 1983, pp. 1312-1318.

Bulkley, B. H. : Salvaging ischemic myocardium after myocardial infarction. Hosp Pract 18, 1983, pp. 61-69.

Cowley, M. J. and Gold, H. K. : Use of intracoronary streptokinase in acute myocardial infarction. Mod Conc Cardiovasc Dis 51, 1982, pp. 97-102.

Furberg, C. D. : Clinical value of intracoronary streptokinase (Editorial). Am J Cardiol 53, 1984, pp. 626-627.

Ganz, W. , Buchbinder, N. , Marcus, H. , Mondkar, A. , Maddahi, J. , Charuzi, Y. , O'Connor, L. , Shell, W. , Fishbein, M. , Kass, R. , Miyamoto, A. , and Swan, J. J. C. : Intracoronary thrombolysis in evolving myocardial infarction. Am Heart J 101, 1981, pp. 4-13.

Ganz, W. , Geft, I. , Maddahi, J. , Berman, D. , Charuzi, Y. , Shah, P. K. , and Swan, H. J. C. : Nonsurgical reperfusion in evolving myocardial infarction. J Am Coll Cardiol 1, 1983, pp. 1247-1253.

Ganz, W. , Geft, I. , Shah, P. K. , Lew, A. S. , Rodriguez, L. ,
Weiss, T. , Maddahi, J. , Berman, D. S. , Charuzi, Y. , and
Swan, H. J. C. : Intravenous streptokinase in evolving myo-
cardial infarction. Am J Cardiol 53, 1984, pp. 1209-1216.

Kennedy, J. W. , Ritchie, J. L. , Davis, K. B. , and Fritz,
J. K. : Western Washington randomized trial of intracoronary
streptokinase in acute myocardial infarction. N Engl J Med
309, 1983, pp. 1477-1482.

Khaja, F. , Walton, J. A. , Jr. , Brymer, J. F. , Lo, E. ,
Osterberger, L. , O'Neill, W. W. , Colfer, H. T. , Weiss, R. ,
Lee, T. , Kurian, T. , Goldberg, A. D. , Pitt, B. , and Goldstein, S. : Intracoronary fibrinolytic therapy in acute myocardial infarction. N Engl J Med 308, 1983, pp. 1305-1311.

Leiboff, R. H. , Katz, R. J. , Wasserman, A. G. , Bren,
G. B. , Schwartz, H. , Varghese, P. J. , and Ross, A. M. : A
randomized, angiographically controlled trial of intracoronary
streptokinase in acute myocardial infarction. Am J Cardiol 53,
1984, pp. 404-407.

Markis, J. E. , Malagold, M. , Parker, J. A. , Silverman,
K. J. , Barry, W. H. , Als, A. V. , Paulin, S. , Grossman, W. ,
and Braunwald, E. : Myocardial salvage after intracoronary
thrombolysis with streptokinase after acute myocardial infarction. N Engl J Med 305, 1981, pp. 777-782.

Mason, D. T. , (Ed.): Proceedings of the Symposium on intracoronary thrombolysis in acute myocardial infarction. Am
Heart J 102, 1981, pp. 1123-1208.

Mason, D. T. and Weinstein, J. (Eds.): Streptokinase thrombolysis in acute myocardial infarction. Am Heart J 104, 1982,
pp. 891-952.

Passamani, E. R. (Ed.): Limitation of Infarct size with
Thrombolytic Agents. Circulation 68 (Part II), 1983, pp.
I-1-I-109.

Rogers, W. J. , Mantle, J. A. , Hood, W. P. , Jr. , Baxley,
W. A. , Whitlow, P. L. , Reeves, R. C. , and Soto, B. :
Prospective randomized trial of intravenous and intracoronary
streptokinase in acute myocardial infarction. Circulation 68,
1983, pp. 1051-1061.

Rude, R. E. , Muller, J. E. , and Braunwald, E. : Efforts to
limit the size of myocardial infarcts. Ann Intern Med 95, 1981,
pp. 736-761.

Schroeder, R. : Systemic versus intracoronary streptokinase
infusion in the treatment of acute myocardial infarction. J Am
Coll Cardiol 1, 1983, pp. 1254-1261.

Spann, J. F. , Sherry, S. , Carabello, B. A. , Denenberg,
B. S. , Mann, R. H. , McCann, W. D. , Gault, J. H. , Gentzler,
R. D. , Belber, A. D. , Maurer, A. H. , and Cooper, E. M. :
Coronary thrombolysis by intravenous streptokinase in acute
myocardial infarction: acute and followup studies. Am J
Cardiol 53, 1984, pp. 655-661.

Stampfer, M. J. , Goldhaber, S. Z. , Yusuf, S. , Peto, R. , and
Hennekens, C. H. : Effect of intravenous streptokinase on acute
myocardial infarction: Pooled results from randomized trials.
N Engl J Med 307, 1982, pp. 1180-1182.

Swan, H. J. C. : Editorial: Thrombolysis in acute myocardial
infarction: Treatment of the underlying coronary artery disease.
Circulation 66, 1982, pp. 914-916.

Swan, H. J. C. : Thrombolysis in acute evolving myocardial
infarction: a new potential for myocardial salvage (Editorial).
N Engl J Med 308, 1983, pp. 1354-1355.

Tennant, S. N. , Dixon, J. , Venable, T. C. , Page, H. L. ,
Jr. , Roach, A. , Kaiser, A. B. , Frederiksen, R. , Tacogue,
L. , Kaplan, P. , Babu, N. S. , Anderson, E. E. , Wooten, E. ,
Jennings, H. S. , III, Breinig, J. , Campbell, W. B. : Intracoronary thrombolysis in patients with acute myocardial
infarction: comparison of the efficacy of urokinase with
streptokinase. Circulation 69, 1984, pp. 754-760.

The International Collaborative Study Group: Reduction of infarct size with the early use of timolol in acute myocardial
infarction. N Engl J Med 310, 1984, pp. 9-15.

Udall, J. A. : Recent advances using streptokinase for acute
coronary thrombosis. Clin Cardiol 7, 1984, pp. 138-147.

VandeWerf, F. , Ludbrook, P. A. , Bergmann, S. R. , Tieten-brunn, A. J. , Fox, K. A. A. , deGeest, H. , Verstraete, M. , Collen, D. , and Sobel, B. E. : Coronary thrombolysis with tissue-type plasminogen activator in patients with evolving myocardial infarction. N Engl J Med 310, 1984, pp. 609-613.

VandeWerf, F. , Bergmann, S. R. , Fox, K. A. A. , deGeest, H. , Hoying, C. F. , Sobel, B. E. , and Collen, D. : Coronary thrombolysis with intravenously administered human tissue-type plasminogen activator produced by recombinant DNA technology. Circulation 69, 1984, pp. 605-610.

ARRHYTHMIAS AND CONDUCTION ABNORMALITIES

Bigger, J. T. , Jr. , Weld, F. M. , and Rolnitzky, L. M. : Which postinfarction ventricular arrhythmias should be treated? Am Heart J 103, 1982, pp. 660-666.

Bigger, J. T. , Jr. , Weld, F. M. , and Rolnitzky, L. M. : Prevalence, characteristics and significance of ventricular tachycardia (three or more complexes) detected with ambu-latory electrocardiographic recording in the late hospital phase of acute myocardial infarction. Am J Cardiol 48, 1981, pp. 815-823.

Carruth, J. E. and Silverman, M. E. : Ventricular fibrillation complicating acute myocardial infarction: Reasons against the routine use of lidocaine. Am Heart J 104, 1982, pp. 545-550.

Chait, L. D. : Management of bradyarrhythmias in acute myo-cardial infarction. Pract Cardiol 7, 1981, pp. 70-79.

Coronary Care Committee of the Council on Clinical Cardiology and the Committee on Medical Education, American Heart Asso-ciation, "Arrhythmias in Acute Myocardial Infarction," Amer-ican Heart Association, Dallas, 1976, p. 109.

Christie, L. G. , Jr. : Lidocaine prophylaxis in acute myo-cardial infarction: expectant or prophylactic use. Pract Cardiol 5, 1979, pp. 37-49.

Hauer, R. N. W. , Lie, K. I. , Liem, K. L. , and Durrer, D. : Long-term prognosis in patients with bundle branch block com-plicating acute anteroseptal infarction. Am J Cardiol 49, 1982, pp. 1581-1585.

Hindman, M. C. , Wagner, G. S. , Taro, M. , Atkins, J. M. ,
Scheinman, M. M. , DeSanctis, R. W. , Hutter, A. H. , Yeatman, L. , Rubenfire, M. , Pujura, C. , Rubin, M. , and
Morris, J. J. : The clinical significance of bundle branch block
complicating acute myocardial infarction. Circulation, 58,
1978, pp. 679-688 and 689-699.

Saksena, S. and Sung, R. J. : The hemiblocks in acute myocardial infarction. Pract Cardiol 6, 1980, pp. 99-122.

Scheinman, M. , Goldschlager, N. , and Peters, R. : Atrioventricular and intraventricular block in patients with acute
myocardial infarction, in Karliner, J. S. and Gregoratos, G.
(Eds.), "Coronary Care," Churchill Livingstone, New York,
1981, pp. 425-448.

HEMODYNAMIC MONITORING

Coronary Care Committee of the Council on Clinical Cardiology
and the Committee on Medical Education, American Heart
Association: "Invasive Techniques for Hemodynamic Measurements," American Heart Association, Dallas, 1973, p. 36.

Forrester, J. S. , Diamond, G. , Chatterjee, K. , and Swan,
H. J. C. : Medical therapy of acute myocardial infarction by
application of hemodynamic subsets. N Engl J Med 295, 1976,
pp. 1356-1362 and 1404-1413.

Gregoratos, G. : Hemodynamic monitoring in the coronary care
unit, in Karliner, J. S. and Gregoratos, G. (Eds.), "Coronary
Care," Churchill Livingstone, New York, 1981, pp. 619-670.

Parmley, W. W. : The post-MI role of hemodynamic monitoring.
Hosp Pract 17, 1982, pp. 169-175.

Swan, H. J. C. and Ganz, W. : Hemodynamic measurements in
clinical practice: A decade in review. J Am Coll Cardiol 1,
1983, pp. 103-113.

CONGESTIVE HEART FAILURE AND
CARDIOGENIC SHOCK

Chatterjee, K. and Parmley, W. W. : Vasodilator therapy
for acute myocardial infarction. J Am Coll Cardiol 1, 1983,
pp. 133-153.

Cohn, J. N.: Vasodilator therapy: Implications in acute myocardial infarction and congestive heart failure. Am Heart J
103, 1982, pp. 773-778.

Fisher, J., Scheidt, S., Collins, M., and Borer, J. S.:
Cardiogenic shock: Pathophysiology and therapy, in Yu, P. N.
and Goodwin, J. F. (Eds.), "Progress in Cardiology," II,
Lea & Febiger, 1982, pp. 163-195.

Gunner, R. F. and Loeb, H. S.: Shock in acute myocardial
infarction: Evaluation of physiologic therapy. J Am Coll
Cardiol 1, 1983, pp. 154-163.

Swan, H. J. C., Shah, P. K., and Rubin, S.: Role of vaso-
dilators in the changing phases of acute myocardial infarction.
Am Heart J 103, 1982, pp. 707-715.

OTHER COMPLICATIONS OF
ACUTE MYOCARDIAL INFARCTION

Bates, R. J., Bentler, S., Resnekov, L., and Anagnostop-
oulous, C. E.: Cardiac rupture: Challenge in diagnosis and
management. Am J Cardiol 40, 1977, pp. 429-437.

Berman, J., Haffajee, C. I., and Alpert, J. S.: Therapy of
symptomatic pericarditis after myocardial infarction: Retrospective and prospective studies of aspirin, indomethacin,
prednisone, and spontaneous resolution, Am Heart J 101, 1981,
pp. 750-753.

Gaudiani, V. A. and Stinson, E. B.: Mechanical defects after
MI: recognition and management. J Cardiovasc Med 8, 1983,
pp. 1265-1273.

Hackel, D. B.: Delayed complications of myocardial infarction. Cardiovasc Rev Rep 3, 1982, pp. 1353-1356.

Kossowsky, W. A., Lyon, A. F., and Spain, D. M.: Re-
appraisal of the postmyocardial infarction Dressler's syndrome. Am Heart J 102, 1981, pp. 954-956.

Loeb, H. S. and Gunnar, R. M.: Management of postinfarction
angina. Pract Cardiol 7, 1981, pp. 39-46.

Marmor, A., Sobel, B. E., and Roberts, R.: Factors pre-
saging early recurrent myocardial infarction ("Extension").
Am J Cardiol 48, 1981, pp. 603-610.

Rackley, C. E. , Russell, R. O. , Mangle, J. A. , Rogers,
W. J. , Papapietro, S. E. , and Schwartz, K. M. : Right ventricular infarction and function. Am Heart J 101, 1981, pp. 215-218.

Radford, M. J. , Johnson, R. A. , Daggett, W. M. , Jr. ,
Fallon, J. T. , Buckley, M. J. , Gold, H. K. , and Leinbach,
R. C. : Ventricular septal rupture: A review of clinical and
physiologic features and an analysis of survival. Circulation
64, 1981, pp. 545-553.

Shabetai, R. : Incidence, significance, and approach to the
diagnosis and therapy of other anatomic and functional sequelae
of acute myocardial infarction, in Karliner, J. S. , and
Gregoratos, G. (Eds.), "Coronary Care," Churchill Livingstone, New York, 1981, pp. 533-558.

PROGNOSIS AFTER MYOCARDIAL INFARCTION

Bulkley, B. H. : Editorial: Site and sequelae of myocardial
infarction. N Engl J Med 305, 1981, pp. 337-338.

DeBusk, R. F. , Kraemer, H. C. , and Nash, E. : Stepwise
risk stratification soon after acute myocardial infarction. Am
J Cardiol, 52, 1983, pp. 1161-1166.

Henning, H. , Gilpin, E. A. , Covell, J. W. , Swan, E. A. ,
O'Rourke, R. A. , and Ross, J. : Prognosis after acute myocardial infarction: A multivariate analysis of mortality and
survival. Circulation, 59, 1979, pp. 1124-1136.

Humphries, J. D. : Survival after myocardial infarction. Mod
Conc Cardiovasc Dis 11, 1977, pp. 51-56.

Hutter, A. M. , DeSanctis, R. W. , Flynn, T. , and Yeatman,
L. A. : Non-transmural myocardial infarction: A comparison
of hospital and late clinical course of patients with that of
matched patients with transmural anterior and transmural inferior myocardial infarction. Am J Cardiol 48, 1981, pp.
595-602.

Madsen, E. B. , Gilpin, E. , Henning, H. , Ahnve, S. , LeWinter,
M. , Ceretto, W. , Joswig, W. , Collins, D. , Pitt, W. , and
Ross, J. , Jr. : Prediction of late mortality after myocardial
infarction from variables measured at different times during
hospitalization. Am J Cardiol 53, 1984, pp. 47-54.

Martin, C. A. , Thompson, P. L. , Armstrong, B. K. ,
Hobbs, M. S. T. , and DeKlerk, N. : Long-term prognosis
after recovery from myocardial infarction: a nine year follow-
up of the Porth Coronary Register. Circulation 68, 1983,
pp. 961-969.

Moss, A. J. : Prognosis after myocardial infarction. Am J
Cardiol 52, 1983, pp. 667-669.

The Multicenter Postinfarction Research Group: Risk stratification and survival after myocardial infarction. N Engl J
Med, 309, 1983, pp. 331-336.

Nasmith, J. , Marpole, D. , Rahal, D. , Homan, J. , Stewart,
S. , and Sniderman, A. : Clinical outcomes after inferior myocardial infarction. Ann Intern Med 96, 1982, pp. 22-26.

Norris, R. M. , Baranaby, P. F. , Brandt, P. W. T. , Geary,
G. G. , Whitlock, R. M. L. , Wild, C. J. , and Barratt-Boyes,
B. G. : Prognosis after recovery from first acute myocardial
infarction: determinants of reinfarction and sudden death.
Am J Cardiol 53, 1984, pp. 408-413.

Rapaport, E. and Remedios, P. : The high risk patient after
recovery from myocardial infarction: Recognition and management. J Am Coll Cardiol 1, 1982, pp. 391-400.

Sanz, G. , Castaner, A. , Betriu, A. , Magrina, J. , Roig, E. ,
Coll, S. , Pare, J. C. , and Navarro-Lopez, F. : Determinants
of prognosis in survivors of myocardial infarction. N Engl J
Med 306, 1982, pp. 1065-1070.

Schuster, E. H. and Bulkley, B. H. : Early postinfarction
angina. Ischemia at a distance and ischemia in the infarct
zone. N Engl J Med 305, 1981, pp. 1101-1105.

Shah, P. K. and Berman, D. S. : Editorial: Implications of
precordial S-T segment depression in acute inferior myocardial
infarction. Am J Cardiol 48, 1981, pp. 1167-1168.

Sniderman, A. D. , Beaudry, J. P. , and Rahal, D. P. : Early
recognition of the patient at late high risk: incomplete infarction and vulnerable myocardium. Am J Cardiol 52, 1983, pp.
669-673.

PREDISCHARGE EXERCISE TESTING

Cohn, P. F.: Current concepts: the role of noninvasive cardiac testing after an uncomplicated myocardial infarction. N Engl J Med 309, 1983, pp. 90-93.

Fuller, C. M., Raizner, A. E., Verani, M. S., Nahormek, P. A., Chahine, R. A., McEntee, C. W., and Miller, R. R.: Early postinfarction treadmill stress testing. Ann Intern Med 94, 1981, pp. 734-739.

Schwartz, K. M., Turner, J. D., Sheffield, L. T., Roitman, D. I., Kansal, S., Papapietro, S. E., Russell, R. O., and Rogers, W. J.: Limited exercise testing soon after myocardial infarction. Ann Intern Med 94, 1981, pp. 727-734.

Stang, T. M. and Lewis, R. P.: Editorial: Early exercise tests after myocardial infarction. Ann Intern Med 94, 1981, pp. 814-815.

Starling, M. R., Crawford, and O'Rourke, R. A.: Treadmill exercise tests predischarge and six weeks post-myocardial infarction to detect abnormalities of known prognostic value. Ann Intern Med 94, 1981, pp. 721-727.

Starling, M. R., Crawford, M. H., Kennedy, G. T., and O'Rourke, R. A.: Superiority of selected treadmill exercise protocols predischarge and six weeks postinfarction for detecting ischemic abnormalities. Am Heart J 104, 1982, pp. 1054-1060.

Theroux, P., Marpole, D. G. F., and Bourassa, M. G.: Exercise stress testing in the post-myocardial infarction patient. Am J Cardiol 52, 1983, pp. 664-667.

Weld, F. M., Chu, K-L., Bigger, J. T., and Rolnitzky, L. M.: Risk stratification with low-level exercise testing 2 weeks after acute myocardial infarction. Circulation 64, 1981, pp. 306-314.

SECONDARY PREVENTION OF MYOCARDIAL INFARCTION

Anturane Reinfarction Trial Policy Committee: The anturane reinfarction trial: Reevaluation of outcome. N Engl J Med 306, 1982, pp. 1005-1008.

Aspirin Myocardial Infarction Study Research Group: A randomized, controlled trial of aspirin in persons recovered from myocardial infarction. JAMA 243, 1980, pp. 661-669.

B-Blocker Heart Attack Trial Research Group: A randomized trial of propranolol in patients with acute myocardial infarction: I. Mortality results. JAMA 247, 1982, pp. 1707-1714.

B-Blocker Heart Attack Trial Research Group: A randomized trial of propranolol in patients with acute myocardial infarction. JAMA 250, 1983, pp. 2814-2819.

E. P. S. I. M. Research Group: A controlled comparison of aspirin and oral anticoagulants in prevention of death after myocardial infarction. N Engl J Med 307, 1982, pp. 701-708.

Frishman, W. H. : Antiplatelet therapy in coronary heart disease. Hosp Prac 17, 1982, pp. 73-86.

Frishman, W. H. , Furberg, C. D. , and Friedewald, W. T. : Drug Therapy: B-adrenergic blockade for survivors of acute myocardial infarction. N Engl J Med 310, 1984, pp. 830-837.

From the N. I. H. : Implications of recent B-blocker clinical trials for patients after myocardial infarction. JAMA 249, 1983, pp. 2482-2483.

Furberg, C. D. , Friedwald, W. T. , and Eberlein, K. A. (Eds.), "Proceedings of the Workshop on Implications of Recent Beta-blocker Trials for Postmyocardial Infarction Patients," Circulation 67 (Part II), 1983, pp. I-1-I-III.

Furberg, C. D. , Hawkins, C. M. , and Lichstein, E. : Effect of propranolol in postinfarction patients with mechanical or electrical complications. Circulation 69, 1984, pp. 761-765.

Hood, W. B. , Jr. : Editorial: More on sulfinpyrazone after myocardial infarction. N Engl J Med 306, 1982, pp. 988-989.

Jones, R. J. : Editorial: β-blockade and recurrent myocardial infarction. JAMA 247, 1982, pp. 2141-2142.

May, G. S. , Furberg, C. D. , Eberlein, K. A. , and Geraci, B. J. : Secondary prevention after myocardial infarction: a review of short-term acute phase trials. Prog Cardiovasc Dis 25, 1983, pp. 335-359.

Moser, M.: Editorial: β -Blockers and myocardial infarction. Arch Intern Med 142, 1982, pp. 1618-1619.

Norwegian Multicenter Study Group: Timolol-induced reduction in mortality and reinfarction in patients surviving acute myocardial infarction. N Engl J Med 304, 1981, pp. 801-807.

Pratt, C. M. and Roberts, R.: Chronic beta blockade therapy in patients after myocardial infarction. Am J Cardiol 52, 1983, pp. 661-664.

Rosman, H. S. and Goldstein, S.: Preventing mortality and morbidity after myocardial infarction. J Cardiovasc Med 7, 1982, pp. 961-966.

Shand, D. G.: Beta-adrenergic blocking drugs after acute myocardial infarction. Mod Conc Cardiovasc Dis 51, 1982, pp. 103-106.

Shand, D. M. (Ed.): "New Perspectives on Beta Blockers in Patients with Acute Myocardial Infarction," Meded, Miami, 1983, p. 45.

Singh, B. N., Phil, D., and Venkatesh, N.: Prevention of myocardial reinfarction and of sudden death in survivors of acute myocardial infarction: role of prophylactic β -adrenoceptor blockade. Am Heart J 107, 1984, pp. 189-200.

Staessen, J., Aulpitt, C., Cattaert, A., VanLees, F. L., and Amery, A.: Editorial: Secondary prevention with beta-adrenoreceptor blockers in post-myocardial infarction patients. Am Heart J 104, 1982, pp. 1395-1399.

Turi, Z. G. and Braunwald, E.: The use of B-blockers after myocardial infarction. JAMA 249, 1983, pp. 2512-2516.

Beta-blockers after myocardial infarction. The Medical Letter, 24, 1982, pp. 43-44.

Chapter 9

CARDIAC REHABILITATION

INTRODUCTION

The transitional period between hospital discharge following myocardial infarction or coronary bypass surgery and return to a full and productive life can be short and smooth or long and difficult. A number of factors influence the rate of recovery, including age, general health, prior activity level, occupation, complicated vs uncomplicated hospital course, and length of hospitalization. A major purpose of cardiac rehabilitation is to ease the transition from the hospital to a normal life by means of an organized program of education, exercise, and psychological support.

THE PURPOSES OF CARDIAC REHABILITATION

1. To improve exercise capacity
2. To increase self-confidence
3. To decrease the frequency of angina attacks
4. To assist in weight control
5. To assist in control of hypertension
6. To assist in control of blood lipids (to increase HDL and to decrease triglycerides, LDL, and VLDL)

ADDITIONAL POSSIBLE BENEFITS OF EXERCISE CONDITIONING PROGRAMS*

1. Improvement in cardiac performance
2. Increase in coronary collateral blood vessels
3. Decrease in cardiac mortality

CANDIDATES FOR A CARDIAC REHABILITATION PROGRAM

1. Patients recovering from acute myocardial infarction
2. Patients recovering from coronary bypass surgery

---

*Unproven, but postulated benefits.

133

3. Patients with stable angina pectoris
4. Patients with stable congestive heart failure due to coronary artery disease
5. Patients who are deconditioned as a result of self- or physician-imposed activity restriction

PATIENTS WHO ARE NOT CANDIDATES FOR EXERCISE PROGRAMS

1. Patients with unstable angina pectoris
2. Patients with severe congestive heart failure
3. Patients with significant arrhythmias
4. Patients with severe hypertension
5. Patients with significant physical impairments
6. Patients with significant peripheral vascular disease (some of these patients may be candidates for a modified exercise conditioning program)

GUIDELINES TO CARDIAC REHABILITATION

1. IN-HOSPITAL PROGRAMS

A great deal can be accomplished by initiating a rehabilitation program early in the course of recovery from acute myocardial infarction or coronary bypass surgery. Particularly important in this phase is the component of education. Patients may have had no previous knowledge of their disease and its implication for their future and may need a great deal of input and reassurance in this regard. Although much of this should come from the patient's physician, this information can be supplemented effectively by cardiac rehabilitation personnel, including nurses, occupational therapists, physical therapists, dieticians, and psychologists. Some hospitals have a fully organized cardiac rehabilitation team including all of these members, while other hospitals can accomplish the same goals with a minimum of specialized personnel. The amount and type of education required varies with the knowledge and sophistication and interest of the individual patient, but virtually all patients will benefit from a program of education. This can be in the form of pamphlets, video cassettes, and organized conferences, or in the form of bedside one-to-one discussions. The subject matter should include the nature of the illness and/or procedures, the short- and long-term modifications in life-style that will be necessary, the purpose and actions of any medications, dietary instructions, activity and exercise instruction, including guidelines for energy conservation. It is particularly

important to be sure the patient is fully informed about all of
these facts at the time of discharge.

The second major component of inpatient cardiac rehabilitation is that of physical conditioning (physical therapy and occupational therapy). A program of physical and occupational
therapy can be initiated during the early recovery phase in the
hospital and advance with the progression of the patient (Table
9-1). The object of this part of the program is to get the patient to the point where he is able to function at home with a
minimum of discomfort and energy dissipation.

2. POSTDISCHARGE CARDIAC REHABILITATION

The education and activity program is begun in the hospital and
continued in the postdischarge period. An important component
of this phase is the predischarge exercise function test (discussed in Chapter 8), which is used to prescribe the activity
level at home as well as to determine the exercise level used
for the rehabilitation program. The maximal MET level
achieved at this test without chest pain, shortness of breath,
fatigue, or signs of ischemia determines how much activity
the patient can safely do at home (Table 9-2).

The maximum heart rate achieved during this test determines the target heart rate for an exercise conditioning program, in that the patient should exercise from 20-30 minutes
at 70-85% of his maximum (safe) heart rate to achieve physical
conditioning (a lower rate may be necessary if the patient has
been started on a beta-blocker drug). The exercise conditioning
program consists of supervised or unsupervised activity, using
any continuous dynamic-type activity that the patient can participate in for 20-30 minutes at a time. Such activities include
walking-jogging (treadmill, track, or any suitable walking
course), bicycling (stationary or standard), rope jumping, or
even such activities as swimming or volleyball. In each case,
the exercise should consist of a 5-10 minute period of calis-
thenic-type warm-ups and 20-30 minutes of dynamic activity,
followed by 5-10 minutes of cool-down activities. Supervised
exercise conditioning programs are usually conducted three
times per week, with the patient supplementing his activity
with walking or bicycling at home several days per week. The
advantages of a supervised program include the ability to
monitor heart rate, arrhythmias, and blood pressure during
and after exercise, as well as to treat arrhythmias, including
defibrillation, which may be necessary on rare occasions. In
addition, the personnel and other patients present provide
information, encouragement, and psychological support, and

Table 9-1. Inpatient Physical and Occupational Therapy in Acute MI

Level	Day	METS*	Physical Therapy	Occupational Therapy
1	1	1	Introduction to program; passive R.O.M. to all extremities.	Introduction to program.
2	1-2	1.5	Active ankle flexion; breathing exercises.	Begin instruction in energy conservation for light self-care.
3	2-3	1.5-2	Active assistance R.O.M. to all extremities.	Monitor performance in light hygiene.
4	3-4	2	Active exercises to all extremities excluding shoulders.	Instruction in bathing, transfer to chair.
5	4-5	2.5	Active exercises to all extremities including shoulders.	Instruction in bathroom transfer.
6	5-6	2.5-3	Increase exercises, add some resistance.	Monitor walking; relaxation training.

7	6-7	3	Sitting and standing warm-up exercises.	Monitor walking in hall; continue education in energy conservation.
8	7-10	3-3.5	Progressive standing warm-up exercises.	Further education in at-home energy conservation, begin education in risk factor modification.
9	10-14	3.5-4	Increase resistive warm-up exercises.	Review discharge instructions.

*1 MET = Energy expenditure at rest; R.O.M. = Range of motion
Compiled from Cardiac Rehabilitation Programs in use at Cedars-Sinai, U. C. L. A. , Brotman and Midway Medical Centers, Los Angeles, CA.

Table 9-2.   Postdischarge Activity Levels

Weeks at Home	METS	Recreational Activities	Work Activities
1-2	1.5-2	Level walking (1 mph); visitors at home.	Desk work, preparing light meals, light housework, business calls.
3-4	2-3	Level walking (2 mph), level bicycling (5 mph); bowling; sexual activities.	Typing, making beds, dining out, light shopping, meal preparations.
5-6	3-4	Level walking (3 mph), level bicycling (6 mph), golf, fishing.	Driving short distances, moderate housework (vacuuming, mopping).
7-8	4-5	Level walking (3.5 mph), level bicycling (8 mph), table tennis, easy dancing, light gardening.	Driving longer distances, heavier housework (cleaning windows, scrubbing floors), air travel.

| 9-10 | 5-6 | Level walking (4 mph), level bicycling (10 mph), swimming, tennis (doubles). | Moderate physical work, digging in garden. |
| 10+ | 6-7 | Level walking (5 mph), bicycling on slopes, tennis (singles). | Moderate to heavy physical work, mowing lawn. |

Compiled from Fox, S. M., Naughton, J. P., and Gorman, P. A.: Physical activity and cardiovascular health. III The exercise prescription; frequency and type of activity. Mod Concepts Cardiovasc Dis 41:6, 1972; and from Zohman, L. R.: Beyond diet.. Exercise your way to fitness and heart health. CPC International 1974; and from Scalzi, C. C.: As the beat goes on. American Heart Association, Greater Los Angeles Affiliate, 1976; and from The approximate metabolic cost of activities. AMSCO Rehab, 1975.

the facility provides the resources and equipment. It may be difficult or inconvenient or even unappealing or too expensive for some patients to participate in such programs, and an unsupervised program is better than no program at all, providing the patient is guided by his physician and takes his pulse during and after activity to determine the appropriate level of activity as well as to monitor for significant arrhythmias. As the exercise program continues over the weeks and months after initiation (the average cardiac rehabilitation program lasts for 3 months, but in some cases it is desirable to continue 4 to 6 months), the level of exercise increases, but the heart rate is still maintained in the 70-85% range. At the end of the cardiac rehabilitation training program, a submaximal exercise stress test is usually performed to see if there is any electrocardiographic or clinical evidence of ischemia at submaximal age-predicted heart rate in order to guide further therapy as well as to determine the safety of higher levels of unsupervised physical activity. It should be emphasized that the completion of a 3- or 4-month cardiac rehabilitation program should not result in cessation of exercise conditioning activities, since this will result in deconditioning and loss of the gain made. It is hoped that patients will have gained the confidence, skills, and desire necessary to continue a life-long program of exercise which will result in improved exercise capacity and lower heart rate and blood pressure response to exercise and possibly lower risks for further cardiac events (discussed further in Chapter 11).

REASONS FOR DROPPING OUT OF A CARDIAC REHABILITATION PROGRAM

Unfortunately, despite the enthusiasm most patients have initially, a significant number either drop out of an organized program before completion or fail to continue an independent program of exercise. In general, this is a result of lack of motivation and interest rather than difficulty or complications resulting from the program. Some of these patients can be induced back into a program with encouragement by physician, family, or friends, but others may be committed to a sedentary life-style. In other cases, patients may have to drop out of a program for medical reasons such as persistent or increasing angina, uncontrolled hypertension, arrhythmias or heart failure, or physical impairments. These patients can often resume a program upon correction or control of these problems.

REFERENCES

American College of Sports Medicine: "Guidelines for Graded Exercise Testing and Exercise Prescription," 2nd Ed. , Lea & Febiger, Philadelphia, 1980.

Brammell, H. L. : Early rehabilitation of the post infarction patient, in Long, C. (Ed.), "Prevention and Rehabilitation in Ischemic Heart Disease," Williams & Wilkins, Baltimore, 1980, pp. 159-185.

Committee on Exercise: "Exercise Testing and Training of Individuals with Heart Disease or at High Risk for its Development: A Handbook for Physicians." American Heart Association, Dallas, 1975.

DeBusk, R. F. : Rehabilitation of the patient soon after myocardial infarction: A physician-oriented approach, in Engelman, K. (Ed.), "Acute Myocardial Infarction: The Post-Hospital Phase," MEDED, Miami, 1982, pp. 35-53.

Froelicher, V. F. and McKirnam, M. D. : Rehabilitation and exercise early after acute myocardial infarction, in Karliner, J. S. and Gregoratus, G. (Eds.), "Coronary Care," Churchill Livingstone, New York, 1981, pp. 897-918.

Murray, G. C. and Beller, G. A. : Cardiac rehabilitation following coronary artery bypass surgery. Am Heart J 105, 1983, pp. 1009-1018.

Robinson, G. , Froelicher, V. F. , and Utley, J. R. : Rehabilitation of the coronary artery bypass graft surgery patient. J Card Rehab 4, 1984, pp. 74-86.

Wenger, N. K. : Rehabilitation of the patient with symptomatic coronary atherosclerotic disease, Baylor College of Medicine, Cardiology Series, p. 3, 1980.

Wenger, N. K. : Rehabilitation of the patient with symptomatic atherosclerotic coronary heart disease, in Hurst, J. W. (Ed.), "The Heart," McGraw-Hill, New York, 1982, pp. 1149-1157.

Wenger, N. K. and Hellerstein, H. K. (Eds.): "Rehabilitation of the Coronary Patient," John Wiley & Sons, Inc. , New York, 1978.

Zohman, L. R. and Kattus, A. A.: Cardiac Rehabilitation For the Practicing Physician, Grune & Stratton, New York, 1979.

Cardiac Rehabilitation Program Guidelines: Cedars-Sinai Medical Center, Brotman Medical Center, Midway Hospital Medical Center and U. C. L. A. Medical Center, Los Angeles, CA.

Chapter 10

CORONARY ARTERY BYPASS SURGERY
AND CORONARY ANGIOPLASTY

INTRODUCTION

Probably no development in cardiology has had as much of an
impact on the therapy of heart disease as has coronary artery
bypass surgery (CABS). Since its development in 1976, over
one million patients have undergone this procedure in the
United States, and the present rate is close to 200,000 operations
per year in this country. As a result of this extensive experience,
a great deal is known about the results of this operation, but
some very fundamental questions still exist regarding the role
of this operation in the treatment of coronary artery disease.
This chapter will discuss the current methods, indications, and
results of this procedure as well as a newer procedure, percutaneous transluminal coronary angioplasty.

TECHNIQUE OF CABS

The principal of CABS is very simple: areas of obstruction
within the coronary arteries (as determined by coronary
arteriography) are bypassed using segments of saphenous
veins taken from the patient and grafted from the ascending
aorta to each diseased coronary artery distal to the site of
obstruction. In some cases, the internal mammary artery
is used to bypass a coronary artery (most often the left anterior
descending vessel) rather than a vein segment, in which case
the origin of the artery from the subclavian artery is left in-
tact but the distal end is ligated and sewn into the coronary
artery. The number of coronary arteries bypassed depends
upon the number of arteries with significant obstructions as
well as the patency of the distal vessels and the viability of
the myocardium, and to a lesser extent, upon the amount of
available vein segments. Thus, the number of bypasses performed on a given patient can be as low as one or as high as
seven or eight (if multiple branches of the major coronary
arteries also have significant lesions) and generally range from

143

two to five per patient. The procedure is performed while the patient is on cardiopulmonary bypass and with the use of a cold, hyperkalemic cardioplegic solution to reduce myocardial oxygen requirements during surgery and thus to preserve myocardial function subsequently. Recently, intraoperative angioplasty has been used in conjunction with CABS in selected patients with multiple serial segmental lesions or with lesions inaccessible to bypass grafting.

Patients usually require an inpatient recuperative period of 7 to 14 days and an outpatient recuperative period which can vary from 3 to 4 weeks to 3 to 6 months before returning to full activity (this period will vary according to age, general physical condition, motivation, and level of activity to be achieved). Patients are started on platelet-inhibiting drugs at the time of surgery. (The optimal combination and dosages are not yet agreed upon, but a common combination is aspirin at a dose of 162 mg/day [2 baby aspirins] and dipyridamadole [Persantine] at a dose of 75 mg t. i. d. , which are continued at least 12 months postoperatively to prevent thrombosis of grafts.)

INDICATION FOR CABS

Current indications for CABS can be divided into the following categories: definite, probable, and possible. In addition, there are a number of situations in which CABS is probably not indicated. These various categories, based on relief of symptoms and/or prolongation of life are outlined as follows:

DEFINITE

1. Patients with stable angina pectoris and multivessel disease whose angina cannot be adequately controlled with medical therapy
2. Patients with unstable angina pectoris and multivessel disease whose angina cannot be adequately controlled medically
3. Patients with a symptomatic and significant ($\geqslant 50\%$) lesion of the left main coronary artery

PROBABLE

1. Patients with symptomatic triple-vessel coronary artery disease with moderate to severe left ventricular dysfunction
2. Patients with symptomatic multivessel disease and indications of being "high risk"

3. Patients with severe ischemic left ventricular dysfunction
4. Asymptomatic patients with severe left main coronary artery disease
5. Patients who have survived primary ventricular fibrillation and have multivessel disease
6. Severely symptomatic patients who have previously undergone CABS and subsequently developed vein graft occlusion or progressive coronary artery disease
7. Patients undergoing other (noncoronary) cardiac surgery who are found to have significant symptomatic or asymptomatic coronary artery disease suitable for CABS

POSSIBLE

1. Mildly to moderately symptomatic patients with three-vessel disease and normal left ventricular function
2. Asymptomatic patients with three-vessel disease
3. Patients with recent myocardial infarction who have indications of being "high risk"

PROBABLY NOT INDICATED

1. Patients with severe left ventricular dysfunction (in the absence of uncontrollable angina)
2. Patients with severe diffuse (distal) coronary disease
3. Patients with mild or absent symptoms and one- or two-vessel disease
4. Patients who could be treated initially with percutaneous transluminal coronary angioplasty (PTCA)
5. Patients at high risk for surgery because of noncardiac reasons

CABS IN STABLE ANGINA PECTORIS

The original indication for performing CABS 15 years ago remains the principal indication today—namely for relief of angina pectoris which is resistant to medical management. CABS is an extremely effective form of therapy for the relief of angina pectoris in patients with suitable coronary anatomy (widely patent vessels distal to a proximal site(s) of obstruction). Angina pectoris is significantly improved in 85-90% of patients undergoing surgery, with 70 to 80% of patients becoming completely asymptomatic. Improvement can be documented objectively by demonstration of increased exercise duration and normal or improved electrocardiographic response to stress testing as well as by reduction in nitroglycerin use. Long-term follow-up has now shown that two-thirds of patients are still improved 8 to 10 years after surgery when compared to their condition prior to surgery, and that close to 50% of patients remain totally asymptomatic. In comparison, only about one-third of patients treated medically over 8 to 10 years show improvement, and only 3% are asymptomatic after the same duration of time.

A less clear-cut indication for surgery is chronic stable angina pectoris with partial response to medical therapy. The decision whether to pursue medical therapy or to recommend surgery in this type of patient is dependent upon several factors, but the primary consideration is usually patient preference. Some patients are very satisfied to live with a certain amount of exercise-induced angina, provided that it does not significantly interfere with their life-style and that the pain is easily relieved with rest and/or nitroglycerin. Other patients would much rather undergo surgery with an acceptably low mortality and morbidity and high likelihood of total or very significant relief of angina pectoris rather than to restrict their activities in order to avoid anginal pains.

A somewhat more difficult question pertains to the management of the patient with easily controlled angina pectoris. In this situation, the mild degree of angina may be due to initially stable and mild angina, or may be a result of mild curtailment of activity, or to successful medical therapy. In any of these cases, the patient is unlikely to opt for surgical therapy unless he is convinced that the surgery will prolong his life or prevent major complications of his disease. The recommendation of surgery for these patients is still controversial and is discussed below.

CABS FOR PROLONGATION OF LIFE
AND PREVENTION OF COMPLICATIONS

Despite 15 years of experience with this operation, the fundamental issue of whether or not CABS prolongs life is still unsettled. Part of the difficulty in answering this question is due to the differences in establishing, maintaining, and interpreting adequately controlled and randomized studies. Also contributing to this problem is the fact that both medical and surgical treatment have advanced considerably in the past 15 years, so that comparisons between medical and surgical therapy applied to patients 10 to 15 years ago may not be valid today. With these reservations in mind, several conclusions have been reached and generally agreed upon as of this date. These conclusions have been drawn from a number of clinical studies utilizing both randomized and nonrandomized methodologies and both angiographic and clinical data.

As of this date, the only uniformly agreed upon indication for surgery in mildly to moderately symptomatic patients with coronary artery disease in order to prolong life is the presence of significant (at least 50%) narrowing of the left main coronary artery. Although isolated left main coronary disease is a relatively uncommon finding in patients with chronic stable angina (occurring in about 5% of such patients), it is particularly lethal, having a mortality of about 9-10% per year. In contrast, the annual mortality of such patients treated with CABS averages only 1-2% per year. The comparable statistics for asymptomatic patients with left main coronary disease are presently unknown, but it is likely that survival would be improved by surgery in this group also.

The concept of "left main equivalent" disease refers to a combination of significant proximal disease of both the left anterior descending and circumflex coronary arteries and was initially felt to carry the same poor prognosis as left main coronary disease. More recent data have shown that the prognosis of patients with this combination is somewhat better than with left main coronary disease but considerably worse than patients with combined lesions with a more distal location in the LAD artery.

There is still disagreement about whether patients with mildly to moderately symptomatic three-vessel coronary artery disease (without left main coronary involvement) have a better survival with surgery compared to medical therapy. Some studies have shown improved survival with surgery in this group of patients as a whole, whereas other studies have shown improved survival only in patients with three-vessel disease and moderately impaired ventricular function (ejection fraction of 30-50%), or even severely impaired ventricular function (ejection fraction less than 30%), and some studies have shown improved survival in patients with three-vessel disease and normal left ventricular function. Differences in survival between medically and surgically treated patients tend to be small, even when significant, averaging only a 2-3% difference per year. The recently published results of the Coronary Artery Surgery Study (CASS), which was a very carefully controlled randomized study with excellent surgical results, included only patients with mild or no angina and excluded ("high risk") patients with unstable angina, congestive heart failure, severe left ventricular dysfunction, or left main coronary artery disease. Five-year survival in both medically and surgically treated groups was excellent (90%) with no significant difference in survival between the groups. (However, almost one-fourth of the patients assigned to the medically treated group switched over to surgical treatment during the five-year period because of symptoms.) This study did not show a trend, however, toward increased survival rate of patients with triple-vessel disease and impaired left ventricular function (LV ejection fraction of 35-50%). In a subgroup of patients not randomized to the study with ejection fractions below 35%, survival was improved in the patients treated surgically, particularly in those with very severe LV dysfunction (ejection fraction below 26%).

Recently, attempts have been made to identify high- and low-risk patients based on clinical and noninvasive criteria in order to better select those patients likely to benefit from surgical therapy. Patients in the high-risk category based on clinical factors (older age, history of congestive heart failure, history of myocardial infarction, history of hypertension, and resting ST segment depression on the electrocardiogram) tend to benefit more from surgical therapy than do patients at low risk. Attempts to identify high-risk patients more accurately by noninvasive techniques, using exercise stress testing or nuclear stress testing, may allow even more accurate identification of patients most likely to benefit from this operation. Such patients would include those with poor exercise tolerance or development of hypotension with exercise, or inability to increase heart rate normally with exercise, as well as those patients with severe and rapid development of ST segment depression and delayed normalization of these abnormalities. Patients who demonstrate a decrease in left ventricular ejection fraction or extensive left ventricular wall motion abnormalities or extensive thallium defects with exercise may also be in this high-risk group.

The effect of surgical therapy on improvement in survival in patients with double-vessel disease is less apparent than with triple-vessel disease, since the natural history of double-vessel disease is more benign than triple-vessel disease. However, high-risk patients, (as defined above) or those with moderately reduced ejection fraction, also appear to have improved survival with surgery when two rather than three vessels are significantly diseased and are suitable for bypass.

Another group of patients who also fit the category of severe double- or triple-vessel disease and who probably are benefited by surgical revascularization include those who develop symptomatic left ventricular dysfunction with ischemic episodes. These patients develop episodes of congestive heart failure or even pulmonary edema as a result of ischemia, rather than as a result of severe fixed left ventricular dysfunction.

One group of patients whose survival is not improved by surgery is the group of patients with single-vessel disease. These patients may have disease limited to the left anterior descending, circumflex, or right coronary artery. As with multivessel disease, such patients may be asymptomatic or mildly, moderately, or severely symptomatic. Regardless of symptoms, survival in these patients appears to be excellent (with the possible exception of patients with high-grade stenosis in the left anterior descending artery proximal to the first septal perforator branch) and is not further improved with surgery. Very symptomatic patients with single-vessel disease may be surgical candidates, however, if their symptoms cannot be controlled adequately with medication. With the development of percutaneous transluminal coronary angioplasty (PTCA), however, this is now the treatment of choice in such patients who are candidates for this procedure (see below).

Another related issue pertains to the prevention of myocardial infarction by CABS. No convincing data have emerged which show that CABS decreases the likelihood of myocardial infarction. In the early experience with this operation, there was significant (15-20%) incidence of perioperative myocardial infarction, thus negating the advantage of a possible later reduction in infarction rate. However, even with the current low perioperative myocardial infarction rate (5%), no reduction in subsequent infarction rate has been demonstrated from CABS in the recent CASS study in a selected population of low-risk patients. Whether CABS can prevent myocardial infarction in a higher-risk group is yet to be determined. One encouraging report recently showed that patients with previous CABS tend to have smaller and less complicated infarctions than other patients.

CABS FOR UNSTABLE ANGINA PECTORIS

As discussed in Chapter 7, the initial management of unstable angina pectoris, whether it is new onset angina, a change in the pattern of stable angina, or postinfarction angina, consists of maximalization of medical therapy, preferably done in the hospital. Most of these patients can have their angina controlled and can be assessed further with electrocardiographic and/or nuclear stress testing and/or coronary arteriography when their condition has stabilized. The decision to operate on these patients is then predicated on the same criteria as in patients with stable angina pectoris. In the small number of patients who do not stabilize in the hospital under maximal medical therapy, however, coronary arteriography is indicated, and coronary bypass surgery is advised if operable two- or three-vessel disease is demonstrated. In the various randomized clinical trials of surgical vs medical therapy for unstable angina pectoris, survival was similar for both groups, but the patients undergoing surgery had less angina subsequently, and many of the patients initially treated medically subsequently required surgery. Although the studies failed to demonstrate improved survival with surgery, it has been concluded, as in the case of stable angina pectoris, that the high-risk subgroup of patients with unstable angina will very likely derive increased survival from CABS. The randomized studies have also failed to demonstrate a decrease in the rate of myocardial infarction in patients treated surgically, but this was largely due to the occurrence of perioperative myocardial infarction, so that the subsequent lower rate of myocardial infarction in the surgical group was offset by the perioperative infarction rate. More recently, with improved surgical technique utilizing myocardial preservation methods, the perioperative myocardial infarction rate has been substantially reduced, so that future comparisons between medical and surgical groups are likely to show a significant reduction in myocardial infarction rate in the surgical patients. A recent, nonrandomized study demonstrated a very low perioperative mortality (1.7%) and excellent 10-year survival rate (83%), without any significant difference in survival between patients with abnormal left ventricular function compared to those with normal ventricular function.

CABS AFTER ACUTE MYOCARDIAL INFARCTION

PATIENTS WITH RECURRENT ANGINA PECTORIS

A significant number of patients with acute myocardial infarction will develop new or recurrent angina pectoris at rest or with minimal activity during their in-hospital recovery period. In many of these patients it will be possible to reduce or eliminate their angina with medical therapy. In others it may be necessary to utilize temporary intraaortic balloon counterpulsation. Patients with refractory postmyocardial infarction angina should be referred for CABS (or PTCA), assuming appropriate anatomy is demonstrated by coronary arteriography. In the remaining patients, whose angina is controlled completely or near completely with medical therapy, subsequent management should be based upon several considerations. It has been determined that as a group, patients with postinfarction angina have a high mortality rate. If these patients are subdivided on the basis of their electrocardiographic pattern during pain, two groups can be defined: those with ischemia in the infarct zone (peri-infarction ischemia) and those with ischemia in an area remote from the acute infarction ("ischemia at a distance"). It has been shown that prognosis is particularly poor (72% 6-month mortality) in patients with ischemia at a distance, compared to patients with ischemia in the infarct zone (33% mortality). It now appears appropriate, therefore, to recommend coronary arteriography in the group of patients with ischemia at a distance during their hospitalization and to proceed with CABS or perhaps PTCA if critical lesions are found in one or more vessels supplying the ischemic area(s). In patients with ischemia in the infarct zone, coronary arteriography is also recommended during initial hospitalization, but the decision to proceed with CABS should be made on an individual basis. In general, such patients will be found to have a subtotal coronary occlusion supplying the area of infarction, with an area of viable but ischemic myocardium surrounding the area of infarction. If severe coronary vessel disease is found in the remaining coronary vessels, CABS is also generally recommended to include all of the vessels with significant disease which are graftable. This approach is particularly recommended in patients with moderate impairment of left ventricular function. Patients with high-grade, single-vessel, subtotal disease with postmyocardial infarction angina should probably be treated with PTCA (see below) if their angina cannot be controlled medically.

PATIENTS WITH REVERSIBLE SEVERE
LEFT VENTRICULAR DYSFUNCTION

In patients who develop severe congestive heart failure (pulmonary edema) with acute myocardial infarction, this may be due to a very large acute myocardial infarction with resultant severe left ventricular dysfunction, or to a combination of new additional left ventricular damage in conjunction with prior left ventricular damage from previous myocardial infarction(s), or to a combination of acute infarction with acute ischemic left ventricular dysfunction. The latter group should also be considered for postmyocardial infarction CABS, since such patients are also at high risk and are probably benefited by surgery. This group of patients may be recognized clinically by transient severe congestive heart failure accompanying acute myocardial infarction, the absence of evidence of extensive myocardial infarction on the electrocardiogram (and frequently the presence of electrocardiographic evidence of ischemia in an area remote from the acute infarction) by only moderate levels of peak CK,

and by the absence of extensive wall motion abnormalities determined by noninvasive nuclear or two-dimensional echo
ventriculography after recovery from acute heart failure. In
contrast, patients with extensive and fixed wall motion abnormalities have a poor prognosis, and ventricular function
and heart failure are unlikely to be helped by CABS unless there
is a discrete left ventricular aneurysm which is felt to be the
basis of heart failure and which is surgically resectable.

CABS IN HIGH-RISK PATIENTS
AFTER ACUTE MYOCARDIAL INFARCTION

The average 1-year mortality following survival from acute
myocardial infarction is 10-15%, with most of these deaths
occurring in the first 6 months. As indicated above, the
mortality is significantly higher in patients with postinfarction
angina. A number of recent studies have shown that patients
can be divided into low- and high-risk groups for subsequent
mortality according to a number of noninvasive as well as invasive indicators (as discussed in Chapter 8). Indicators of
high risk include older age, anterior myocardial infarction
(subendocardial, or "non-transmural" myocardial infarction
is associated with a low in-hospital mortality but a high subsequent mortality), prior myocardial infarction, congestive
heart failure, conduction defects, poor left ventricular function
(ejection fraction of less than 50% and especially an ejection
fraction of less than 30%), the presence of complex ventricular
arrhythmias during the inpatient convalescent period (especially
in the presence of abnormal left ventricular function), and an
abnormal response to low-level exercise testing within 3 weeks
after acute infarction (see Chapter 8). The development of an
ischemic electrocardiographic response to a low level of exercise, with or without the development of angina, is associated
with an approximately 10-fold higher risk of mortality compared to patients without an ischemic response (20% vs 2%). It
is generally felt, therefore, that patients with an ischemic
response to low-level exercise should have elective coronary
arteriography and should be considered for CABS if there is
multivessel coronary artery disease, especially in conjunction
with moderate impairment of left ventricular function.
    Although several studies have shown no increased survival
in asymptomatic postmyocardial infarction patients treated
surgically, most of these patients were in a low-risk category
to begin with. Another study has shown improved survival in
postmyocardial infarction patients treated surgically in a group
of patients with a moderate to large area of myocardium at risk,

defined by the presence of a significant amount of normally contracting left ventricular myocardium supplied by stenotic coronary arteries. The 2-year survival in this surgical sub-group was 93% compared to 64% in the subgroup managed medically. One way to identify such patients would be by routine angiography in all postmyocardial patients who are otherwise suitable for CABS, and this approach is recommended and followed by a number of cardiologists. However, it is likely that high-risk patients who would benefit from surgery can be recognized by noninvasive means utilizing the pre-discharge low-level exercise test and, if necessary, a higher level exercise nuclear stress test at a later phase of con-valescence. As in the case of stable angina, patients who show significant wall motion abnormalities with exercise (outside the area of recent myocardial infarction), particularly when associated with a fall in ejection fraction, are likely to be at high risk and are likely to benefit from CABS. Similarly, patients who develop estensive and reversible thallium defects with exercise, remote from the area of myocardial infarction, are also likely to fall into a high-risk category and should be considered for angiography and CABS.

An overall strategy for the approach to the patient following acute myocardial infarction, is summarized in Figure 10-1.

CABS IN CONJUNCTION WITH OTHER CARDIAC SURGERY IN THE ACUTE MYOCARDIAL INFARCTION PATIENT

As described in Chapter 8, patients who develop "mechanical" complications of acute myocardial infarction leading to heart failure such as ruptured ventricular septum, papillary muscle, chordae tendinae, or ventricular free wall, require surgery to correct the complication and usually undergo CABS at the same time, if possible. If there is single-vessel disease and no viable myocardium is felt to be remaining distal to the obstruction, there is probably no justification in performing CABS at the time. However, if there is multivessel disease and viable myo-cardium distal to the partially or totally obstructive lesion, then it seems reasonable to perform CABS in conjunction with the other surgery, even if ischemia has not been demonstrated.

CABS IN SURVIVORS OF SUDDEN DEATH

It has been shown that most patients who survive an episode of "sudden death" (presumably due to ventricular fibrillation) have not suffered from an acute myocardial infarction but do usually

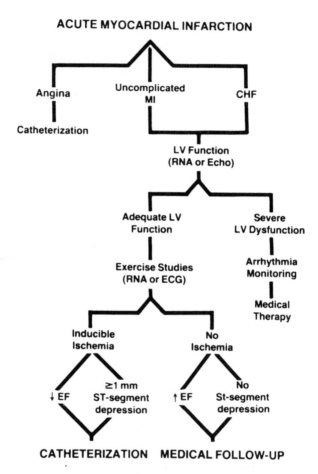

Figure 10-1.   Strategy for identification of patients who should undergo cardiac catheterization after acute myocardial infarction (see text for discussion). (Reprinted by permission from: Epstein, S. E., Palmeri, S. T., and Patterson, R. E.: Current concepts: Evaluation of patients after acute myocardial infarction: Indications for cardiac catheterization and surgical intervention. N Engl J Med 307, 1982, p. 1491.)

have severe triple-vessel or left main coronary artery disease and are subject to recurrent episodes of ventricular fibrillation. The presumption has been made that the episodes of ventricular fibrillation are most likely due to severe ischemia. It has therefore been recommended that all patients who survive primary ventricular fibrillation (i. e. , not associated with acute myocardial infarction) should undergo diagnostic coronary arteriography. If left main or severe three-vessel disease is demonstrated, CABS should be performed. It is not known whether this approach prevents recurrent episodes of ventricular fibrillation and sudden death but it has been shown by several groups that patients with coronary artery disease who have had CABS have a lower incidence of sudden death compared to patients with coronary artery disease treated medically. Whether CABS is an equally or more effective preventative form of therapy than is antiarrhythmic therapy in high-risk patients is still unknown. Although it has been shown that CABS, with or without associated left ventricular aneurysm resection or infarctectomy, has been effective in reducing the frequency of malignant ventricular arrhythmias in selected patients, CABS is not felt to be generally effective in the treatment of ventricular arrhythmias except when due to ischemia.

CABS IN PATIENTS WITH PRIOR CABS

As discussed below, there is a significant incidence of recurrence of angina after CABS. This may be due to early graft closure, to late graft closure, or to progressive coronary artery disease in ungrafted vessels or in grafted vessels distal to the site of graft implantation. The indications for repeat CABS are essentially the same as for initial CABS, although the surgery is technically more difficult and usually patients are less willing to undergo repeat surgery. If early graft closure was due to an avoidable technical surgical problem, there should in general be no reluctance to recommend repeat surgery, even at a short interval after the first operation. If early graft closure is felt to be on the basis of a poor vein used for the graft, it may be possible to do the repeat surgery with an internal mammary graft, which has a longer patency than vein grafts. If, on the other hand, early graft closure was due to diffuse distal coronary disease (poor run-off), it is unlikely that repeat surgery will be any more successful. Overall results in terms of operative mortality, perioperative infarction, graft patency, and survival for repeat CABS are similar to results of initial surgery, although relief of angina is somewhat less common with repeat surgery. An alternative to reoperation in selected patients, is PTCA, which is discussed later.

CABS IN CONJUNCTION WITH
OTHER CARDIOVASCULAR SURGERY

Another indication for CABS is in patients undergoing noncoronary surgery (such as valve replacement) in whom
significant coronary artery lesions have been demonstrated
by coronary arteriography done at the time of cardiac catheterization. It is generally felt that CABS should be done to
all significantly diseased arteries at the time of valve replacement, even in the absence of symptoms or evidence of ischemia.
By such preventive surgery, it is felt that perioperative and
subsequent mortality will be reduced due to prevention of
ischemia and infarction.

A more complicated issue is the use of CABS in conjunction
with cerebrovascular or peripheral vascular disease. There
is a very high association of coronary artery disease with
cerebrovascular and peripheral vascular disease, and it has
been recognized that perioperative and late mortality in patients
undergoing surgery for vascular disease is usually due to
complications of the coexisting coronary disease. Therefore,
it is recommended that patients undergoing elective vascular
surgery be evaluated preoperatively for evidence of coronary
disease, including treadmill testing if feasible. If on the basis
of clinical evaluation and/or noninvasive testing, there is suspicion of severe coronary disease, coronary arteriography
should be done if feasible. Depending upon the relative severity
of the vascular disease compared to the coronary disease, as
well as the urgency of the operation for the vascular problem,
several approaches are possible. If the coronary disease is not
felt to be critical, based on clinical and perhaps noninvasive or
angiographic evidence, and the patient is asymptomatic or mildly symptomatic from the coronary disease, the vascular surgery
can usually be done without associated coronary surgery. If,
on the other hand, the coronary disease is very severe, or the
patient is very symptomatic from the coronary disease, CABS
should generally precede the vascular procedure. In cases of
equally severe carotid and coronary disease, it is often preferable to do both operations simultaneously.

COMPLICATIONS OF CABS

Operative mortality in most hospitals is now in the range of
1-2%, with slightly higher mortality in patients over age 65
(about 5%), in females, and in patients with subtotal left main
coronary disease, as well as in patients with significant left
ventricular dysfunction and in those patients operated upon

emergently. The most frequent nonfatal complication is peri-operative myocardial infarction. This complication is currently estimated to occur in about 5% of patients (one recent report quoted only a 1.5% rate) and is slightly higher in patients with unstable angina pectoris (10%). Other complications of CABS include reoperation for bleeding (incidence about 2.5%), cerebro-vascular accidents (frequency of 1-2% with half of the events being transient), and wound infection or dehiscence (1-5%). Other less serious complications include atrial and ventricular arrhyth-mias, conduction defects, pericarditis (postpericardiotomy syn-drome), "pump" (left ventricular) failure, aortic dissection, bleeding disorders, and cytomegalic virus (CMV) infection, which are all potentially serious but infrequent complications of CABS.

Graft occlusion after CABS is also a complication and often results in recurrence of angina. This can occur early (usually within the first 6 months), in which case it is almost always due either to technical problems or to thrombosis in the graft. The latter is more frequent in vein grafts of small diameter and in those with low flow rates as well as in grafts supplying vessels in which endarterectomies were also done. The incidence of early vein graft thrombosis has been significantly reduced (from 30% to 10%) with the early use of agents which interfere with platelet function (aspirin and dipyridamole). One-year vein graft patency is now 85-90%, and 1-year patency rate for internal mammary grafts is about 95%. Late vein graft closure is due either to intimal hyperplasia or to arteriosclerosis within the graft. At 5 years after surgery, 80-85% vein grafts remain patent, and by 10 to 12 years, there is about 65% patency, with the lowest occlusion rate in left anterior descending grafts. Recurrence of angina after successful bypass surgery is about 5% per year, as a result of either vein graft occlusion or pro-gression of coronary artery disease. Despite this, it has been estimated that only 7% of patients will need reoperation within 10 years.

Five-year survival after CABS for three-vessel disease done in the past 10 years has been 90%, with 93% and 97% survival in patients with double- and single-vessel disease respectively, with only slightly reduced survival in patients with moderately abnormal left ventricular dysfunction, but significantly reduced survival in patients with severe left ventricular dysfunction. Ten-year overall survival after CABS is now about 70%.

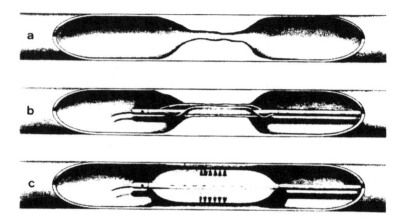

Figure 10-2. Technique of percutaneous transluminal coronary angioplasty. (a) diagrammatic representation of an area of stenosis within a coronary artery. (b) the position of the dilating balloon catheter across the lesion prior to inflation. (c) inflation of the balloon, resulting in enlargement of the lumen. (Reprinted with permission from: Gruntzig, A. R. , Senning, A. , and Siegenthaler, W. E. : Nonoperative dilatation of coronary-artery stenosis. Percutaneous transluminal coronary angioplasty. N Engl J Med 301, 1979, p. 62.)

PERCUTANEOUS TRANSLUMINAL ANGIOPLASTY (PTCA)

Since 1977 a new therapeutic option has been available for the treatment of coronary artery disease by means of nonsurgical revascularization. This technique is known as percutaneous transluminal coronary angioplasty (PTCA) and is a modification of the technique originally developed for use in peripheral vascular disease (Figure 10-2).

METHOD

The procedure is done in the cardiac catheterization laboratory with the cardiac surgery team and operating room on standby. PTCA is accomplished through the use of a specially designed catheter with an inflatable balloon near the tip and a separate lumen for monitoring proximal and distal intracoronary pressure.

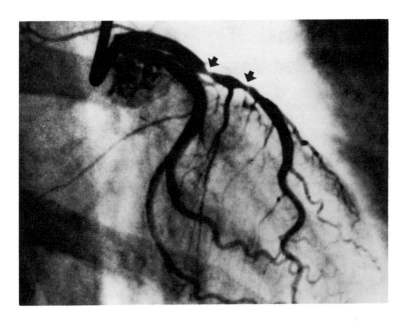

Figure 10-3A. Cineangiographic frames, before (a), during (b), and following (c) successful PTCA of two high-grade sequential lesions (arrows) in a left anterior descending coronary artery. Frame (b) shows the inflated balloon across the lesions. (Courtesy of Simon H. Stertzer, M. D.)

A special guiding coronary angiography catheter, similar to a standard coronary angiography catheter, is first introduced into the ascending aorta by either the femoral or brachial approach and then introduced into the ostium of the appropriate coronary artery. The lesion to be dilated is identified by injection of contrast material through this catheter (Figure 10-3A), and the dilating (balloon) catheter is then inserted through the guiding catheter and advanced into the coronary artery under fluoroscopy. The narrowed segment is crossed with this catheter and the balloon is positioned in the segment to be dilated (Figure 10-2B). Intracoronary pressure is then recorded proximally and distally to the obstruction, with the difference in pressure corresponding to the degree of obstruction. The balloon is then inflated (Figures 10-2C and 10-3B) with a mixture of radiographic contrast material and saline to a pressure of 8-15 atmospheres for 30-60 seconds and then deflated. Repeat proximal and distal intracoronary pressures and selective angiography are performed to evaluate the success of the

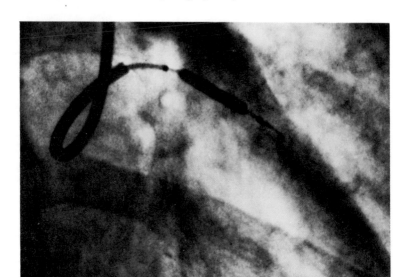

Figure 10-3B.

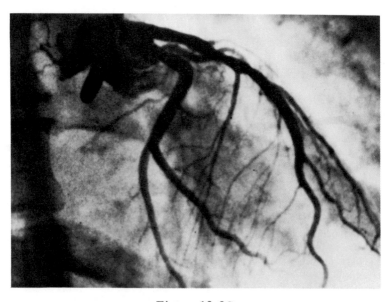

Figure 10-3C.

procedure, and repeat dilatations are performed up to several more times if necessary. Repeat pressure measurements after successful dilatation should show nearly complete obliteration of the pressure gradient across the lesion, and angiography should show significant increase in lumen size (Figure 10-3C). Following the procedure, the catheters are withdrawn, and the patient can be discharged in 1 to 2 days. The procedure is done while the patient is receiving heparin, as well as low molecular weight dextran and platelet inhibitors, and the latter drugs (aspirin and dipyridamole) are continued for 6 months after the procedure to prevent thrombosis, and a calcium channel blocking drug is given to prevent spasm.

INDICATIONS

DEFINITE

1. Patients with severe angina pectoris with a single high-grade proximal or midcoronary stenosis which is concentric, short, and noncalcified (other than left main coronary artery lesions)
2. Patients who previously have undergone successful PTCA and subsequently develop symptomatic restenosis at the same site

PROBABLE

1. Symptomatic patients with sequential coronary lesions in a single coronary vessel, all of which are dilatable
2. Symptomatic patients with a slightly eccentric, high-grade single coronary lesion
3. Symptomatic patients with multivessel coronary artery disease in whom only one of the coronary arteries contains a high-grade lesion which is suitable for dilatation
4. Symptomatic patients with multivessel coronary disease who are not suitable for CABS because of high risk due to cardiac or other medical problems and have lesions suitable for PTCA
5. Symptomatic patients with previous CABS with high-grade stenosis of the distal vein graft at the anastomosis of the coronary artery
6. Symptomatic patients with recent (maximum of a few weeks) total occlusion of a single proximal coronary artery

POSSIBLE

1. Mildly to moderately symptomatic patients with a dilatable single-vessel lesion
2. Asymptomatic patients with a high-grade, single-vessel dilatable lesion with objective evidence of significant ischemia
3. Symptomatic patients with previous CABS with a dilatable lesion in the body of the bypass graft
4. Symptomatic patients with double- or triple-vessel disease with lesions suitable for dilatation in more than one vessel, who are also suitable candidates for CABS
5. Patients with acute myocardial infarction, following successful streptokinase treatment, in whom there is a high-grade dilatable lesion

CONTRAINDICATED

1. Patients with left main coronary artery disease
2. Patients who refuse consent for CABS (with some specific exceptions)
3. Patients with calcified, very eccentric, or very long lesions or with lesions in portions of the coronary arteries inaccessible to a dilating catheter
4. Patients with lesions involving the origin of one or more significant branch vessels

Using the above criteria, it is estimated at the present time that only 5-10% of patients undergoing coronary angiography for consideration of CABS are definite candidates for PTCA, although with increased experience with this technique, the indications may become liberalized. Since in a small percentage of patients (see below), emergency CABS may be necessary following unsuccessful attempts at PTCA, most patients considered for PTCA should also be candidates for CABS and should be prepared (physically and mentally) for this possibility at the time of PTCA.

RESULTS

As is probably true for all procedures which require skill and experience, it has been clearly shown that the success rate is directly proportional and the complication rate indirectly proportional to the experience of the personnel performing the procedure. In the multicenter National Heart, Lung and Blood Institute study involving over 3,000 patients between 1977 and

1981, the primary success rate for PTCA (in which 73% of patients had single-vessel disease) was only 55%, but in the last 2 years of the study, the overall success rate was 70%, with individual hospitals reporting success rates varying from 50-90% according to experience. The highest success rate is seen in patients who have lesions dilated in the left anterior descending artery, with lesser success rates in the right coronary artery and in the circumflex artery. Most failures to successfully dilate a vessel occurred because of inability to reach or cross the stenotic segment with a dilating catheter. (With the recent introduction of steerable dilating catheters, the success rate has been much higher.) The remaining failures resulted from inability to successfully dilate the lesion. Of the patients who have a successful anatomic result, virtually 100% have immediate improvement in angina, and 80% remain stable over the first 3 years, with approximately 50% being asymptomatic at 3 years. Improvement in exercise performance, in left ventricular function and thallium perfusion, as well as improvement in symptoms have been well documented following this procedure. Recently, data with multivessel dilatations have also shown results comparable to single-vessel dilatation, when patients are carefully selected.

Approximately 20-25% patients redevelop stenosis at the site of the angioplasty within 6 months and require repeat PTCA. Of interest and importance, the immediate and late success rate of repeat PTCA exceeds that of initial PTCA. A higher restenosis rate of about 50% is seen in dilatations of the proximal portion or body of stenosed vein grafts, compared with only about a 20% restenosis rate when dilatations are done in the distal vein graft at the site of anastomosis with the coronary artery.

COMPLICATIONS

The most frequent complication is arterial dissection (9%) with or without complete occlusion of the vessel. In the multicenter NHLBI study, 5% of patients had an acute myocardial infarction as a result of the procedure and 6.6% of patients required emergency CABS, with a total mortality of 0.9%. In recent data from a center with a vast experience, only 1.7% of patients had acute myocardial infarction, 3.7% required emergency CABS, and mortality was only 0.01%. No differences in complications and mortality were noted in patients with single-vessel disease or multivessel disease in whom one vessel was dilated, and more recent data suggest that the complication and mortality rate is similar in carefully selected patients in whom multiple vessels are dilated. The highest complication rates were seen in patients with unstable angina pectoris and in patients with very tight (greater than 90%) lesions with unsuccessful dilatation and in the hands of persons with less experience.

REFERENCES

CORONARY ARTERY BYPASS SURGERY

GENERAL INDICATIONS AND RESULTS

Alderman, E. L. , Fisher, L. D. , Litwin, P. , Kaiser, G. C. , Myers, W. O. , Maynard, C. , Levine, F. , and Schloss, M. : Results of coronary artery surgery in patients with poor left ventricular function (CASS). Circulation 68, 1983, pp. 785-795.

Berkoff, H. A. : Management of coronary artery and peripheral vascular disease combinations: a surgeon's view. Council on Cardiology Newsletter, 9, 1983, pp. 1-9.

Braunwald, E. : Effects of coronary-artery bypass grafting on survival. Implications of the randomized Coronary-Artery Surgery Study (Editorial). N Engl J Med 309, 1983, pp. 1181-1184.

Brundage, B. , Massie, B. M. , and Botvinick, E. H. : Improved regional ventricular function after successful surgical revascularization. J Am Coll Cardiol 3, 1984, pp. 902-908.

Campeau, L. , Enjalbert, M. , Lesperance, J. , Vaislic, C. , Grondin, C. M. , and Bourassa, M. G. : Atherosclerosis and late closure of aortocoronary saphenous vein grafts: sequential angiographic studies at 2 weeks, 1 year, 5 to 7 years, and 10 to 12 years after surgery. Circulation, 68, Suppl. II, 1983, pp. II-1-7.

Carr, K. W. , Engler, R. L. , and Ross, J. Jr. : Do coronary artery bypass operations prolong life? West J Med 136, 1982, pp. 295-308.

CASS principle investigators and their associates: Coronary Artery Surgery Study (CASS): a randomized trial of coronary artery bypass surgery. Survival data. Circulation, 68, 1983, pp. 939-950.

CASS principle investigators and their associates: Coronary Artery Surgery Study (CASS): a randomized trial of coronary artery bypass surgery. Quality of life in patients randomly assigned to treatment groups. Circulation, 68, 1983, pp. 951-960.

CASS principle investigators and their associates: Myocardial infarction and mortality in the Coronary Artery Surgery Study (CASS) randomized trial. N Engl J Med 310, 1984, pp. 750-758.

Chaitman, B. R. , Fisher, L. D. , Aourassa, M. G. , Davis, K. , Rogers, W. J. , Maynard, C. , Tyras, D. H. , Berger, R. L. , Judkins, M. P. , Ringqvist, I. , Mock, M. B. , Killip, T. , and participating CASS medical centers: Effect of coronary bypass surgery on survival patterns in subsets of patients with left main coronary artery disease. Report of the collaborative study in coronary artery surgery (CASS). Am J Cardiol 48, 1981, pp. 765-777.

Chaitman, B. R. , Davis, K. , Fisher, L. D. , Bourassa, M. G. , Mock, M. B. , Lesperance, J. , Rogers, W. J. , Fray, D. , Tyras, D. H. , Judkins, M. P. , Ringqvist, I. , Killip, T. , and participating CASS hospitals: A life table and Cox regression analysis of patients with combined proximal left anterior descending and proximal left circumflex coronary artery disease: non-left main equivalent lesions (CASS). Circulation 68, 1983, pp. 1163-1170.

Chesebro, T. H. , Fuster, V. , Elveback, L. R. , Clements, I. P. , Smith, H. P. , Holmes, D. R. , Jr. , Bardsley, W. T. , Pluth, J. R. , Wallace, R. B. , Puga, F. J. , Orszulak, T. A. , Piechler, T. M. , Danielson, G. K. , Schaff, H. V. , and Frye, R. L. : Effect of dipyridamole and aspirin on late vein-graft patency after coronary bypass operations. N Engl J Med 310, 1984, pp. 209-214.

Cooley, D. A. , Hall, R. J. , Elayda, M. A. , Gray, A. G. , and Mathur, V. S. : Aortocoronary bypass surgery: Long term followup of 21,561 patients over one decade (Abstr.). Circulation 66, 1982, Part II, pp. II-219.

Detre, K. M. , Peduzzi, P. , Hammermeister, K. E. , Murphy, M. L. , Hultgren, H. N. , Takaro, T. , and the participants of the Veterans Administration Cooperative Study for Surgery for Coronary Artery Occlusive Disease: Five-year effect of medical and surgical therapy on resting left ventricular function in stable angina: Veterans Administration Cooperative Study. Am J Cardiol 53, 1984, pp. 444-450.

Frye, R. L. and Frommer, P. L. (Eds.): Consensus development conference on coronary artery bypass surgery: Medical and scientific aspects. Circulation 65, Part II, pp. II-1-II-129.

Gersh, B. J., Kronmal, R. A., Frye, R. L., Schaff, H. V., Ryan, T. J., Gosselin, A. J., Kaiser, G. C., Killip, T. III, and participants in the Coronary Artery Surgery Study: Coronary arteriography and coronary artery bypass surgery: Morbidity and mortality in patients ages 65 or older. A report from the Coronary Artery Surgery Study. Circulation 67, 1983, pp. 483-491.

Gitler, B.: Efficacy of antiplatelet drugs in the maintenance of aortocoronary vein bypass graft patency. Am Heart J 106, 1983, pp. 563-570.

Hall, R. J., Elayda, M. A., Gray, A., Mathur, V. S., Garcia, E., DeCastro, C. M., Massumi, A., and Cooley, D. A.: Coronary artery bypass: long-term followup of 22,284 consecutive patients. Circulation 68, Part II, 1983, pp. II-20-26.

Hurst, J. W.: The "overshadowed" CASS report. (Editorial). Clin Cardiol 7, 1984, pp. 193-197.

La Follette, L., Jacobson, L. B., and Hill, J. D.: Isolated aortocoronary bypass operations in patients over 70 years of age - a comparison with results in patients 50 to 59 years old. West J Med 133, 1980, pp. 15-18.

Lawrie, G. M., Morris, G. C., Calhoon, J. H., Safi, H., Zamora, J. L., Beltengady, M., Baron, A., Silvers, A., and Chapman, D. W.: Clinical results of coronary bypass in 500 patients at least 10 years after operation. Circulation 66, 1982, Suppl. I., pp. I-1-I-5.

Lawrie, G. M. and Morris, G. C. Jr.: The role of surgery in the treatment of coronary artery disease: surgical prospective. Baylor College of Medicine Cardiology Series, 6, 1983, pp. 6-27.

Loop, F. D., Sheldon, W. C., Lytle, B. W., Cosgrove, D. M. III, and Proudfit, W. L.: The efficacy of coronary surgery. Am Heart J 101, 1981, pp. 86-95.

Loop, F. D. , Golding, L. R. , MacMillan, J. P. , Cosgrove, D. M. , Lytle, B. W. , and Sheldon, W. C. : Coronary artery surgery in women compared with men: Analysis of risks and long-term results. J Am Coll Cardiol 1, 1983, pp. 383-390.

Mathur, V. S. and Guinn, G. A. : Prospective randomized study to evaluate coronary bypass surgery: 10 year follow-up (Abstr). Circulation 66, 1982, Part II, pp. II-219.

Miller, D. W. , and Ivey, T. D. : Selection of patients for coronary bypass operations. West J Med 133, 1980, pp. 210-217.

Pigott, T. D. , Kouchoukos, N. T. , Oberman, A. , and Cutter, G. : Late results of medical and surgical therapy for patients with coronary artery disease and depressed ejection fraction (Abstr.). Circulation 66, 1982, Part II, pp. II-220.

Rahimtoola, S. H. : Coronary bypass surgery for chronic angina - 1981. A perspective. Circulation 65, 1982, 225-241.

Shark, W. M. and Kass, R. M. : Repeat myocardial revascularization in coronary disease therapy: Consideration of primary bypass failure and success of second graft surgery. Am Heart J 102, 1981, pp. 303-307.

Waters, D. D. , Pelletier, G. B. , Hache, M. , Theroux, P. , and Campeau, L. : Myocardial infarction in patients with previous coronary bypass surgery. J Am Coll Cardiol 3, 1984, pp. 909-915.

Weiner, D. A. , Ryan, T. J. , McCabe, C. H. , Chaitman, B. R. , Sheffield, L. T. , Ferguson, T. C. , Fisher, L. D. , and Tristani, F. : Prognostic importance of a clinical profile and exercise test in medically treated patients with coronary artery disease. J Am Coll Cardiol 3, 1984, pp. 772-779.

CABS FOR UNSTABLE ANGINA PECTORIS

Brown, C. A. , Hutter, A. M. , DeSanctis, R. W. , Gold, H. K. , Leinbach, R. C. , Roberts-Niles, A. , Austen, W. G. , and Buckley, M. T. : Prospective study of medical and urgent surgical therapy in randomizable patients with unstable angina pectoris: Results of in-hospital and chronic mortality and morbidity. Am Heart J 102, 1981, pp. 959-964.

Hultgren, H. N. , Shettigar, U. R. , and Miller, D. C. : Medical versus surgical treatment of unstable angina. Am J Cardiol 80, 50, 1982, pp. 663-670.

Rahimtoola, S. H. , Nunley, D. , Grunkemeier, G. , Tepley, T. , Lambert, L. , and Starr, A. : Ten-year survival after coronary bypass surgery for unstable angina. N Engl J Med 308, 1983, pp. 676-681.

Unstable angina pectoris: National cooperative study to compare medical and surgical therapy. II. In-hospital experience and initial follow-up results in patients with one, two, and three vessel disease. Am J Cardiol 42, 1978, pp. 839-848.

Unstable angina pectoris: National cooperative study to compare medical and surgical therapy. IV. Results in patients with left anterior descending coronary artery disease. Am J Cardiol 48, 1981, pp. 517-524.

CABS AFTER ACUTE MYOCARDIAL INFARCTION

Epstein, S. E. , Palmeri, S. T. , and Patterson, R. E. : Current concepts: Evaluation of patients after acute myocardial infarction: indications for cardiac catheterization and surgical intervention. N Engl J Med 307, 1982, pp. 1487-1492.

Gray, R. J. , Sethna, D. , and Matloff, J. M. : The role of cardiac surgery in acute myocardial infarction. I. With mechanical complications. Am Heart J 106, pp. 723-728.

Gray, R. J. , Sethna, D. , and Matloff, J. M. : The role of cardiac surgery in acute myocardial infarction. II. Without mechanical complications. Am Heart J 106, pp. 728-735.

Norris, R. M. , Agnew, T. M. , Brandt, P. W. T. , Graham, K. J. , Hill, D. G. , Kerr, A. R. , Lowe, J. B. , Roche, A. G. H. , Whitlock, R. M. L. , and Barratt-Boyes, B. G. : Coronary surgery after recurrent myocardial infarction: Progress of a trial comparing surgical with nonsurgical management for asymptomatic patients with advanced coronary disease. Circulation 63, 1981, pp. 785-792.

Rapaport, E. and Remedios, P. : The high risk patient after recovery from myocardial infarction: Recognition and management. J Am Coll Cardiol 1, 1983, pp. 391-400.

Rogers, W. J. , Smith, L. R. , Oberman, A. , Kouchoukas, N. T. , Mantle, J. A. , Russell, R. O. , and Rackley, C. E. : Coronary revascularization surgery. Feasibility after myocardial infarction. Postgrad Med 69, 1981, pp. 36-49.

Sanz, G. , Custaner, A. , Betrin, A. , Magrina, J. , Roig, E. , Coll, S. , Pare, J. C. , and Navarro-Lopez, F. : Determinants of prognosis in survivors of myocardial infarction: A prospective clinical angiographic study. N Engl J Med 306, 1982, pp. 1065-1070.

Schuster, E. H. and Bulkley, B. H. : Early post-infarction angina: Ischemia at a distance and ischemia in the infarct zone. N Engl J Med 305, 1981, pp. 1101-1105.

PERCUTANEOUS TRANSLUMINAL
CORONARY ANGIOPLASTY (PTCA)

Block, P. C. : Percutaneous transluminal angioplasty, in Yu, P. N. and Goodwin, J. F. (Eds.), "Progress in Cardiology," Vol. 11, Lea & Febiger, Philadelphia, 1982, pp. 1-18.

Block, P. C. , Cowley, M. J. , Kaltenbach, M. , Kent, K. M. , and Simpson, J. : Percutaneous angioplasty of stenosis of bypass grafts or of bypass graft anastomotic sites. Am J Cardiol 53, 1984, pp. 566-568.

Council on Scientific Affairs: Percutaneous transluminal angioplasty. JAMA 251, 1984, pp. 764-768.

Cowley, M. J. and Block, P. C. : Percutaneous transluminal angioplasty. Mod Conc Cardiovasc Dis 50, 1981, pp. 25-29.

Dorros, G. , Cowley, M. J. , Simpson, J. , Bentivoglio, L. G. , Block, P. C. , Bourassa, M. , Detre, K. , Gosselin, A. J. , Gruntzig, A. , Kelsey, S. F. , Kent, K. M. , Mock, M. B. , Mullin, S. M. , Myler, R. K. , Passamani, E. R. , Stertzer, S. H. , and Williams, D. O. : Percutaneous transluminal coronary angioplasty: Report of complications from the National Heart, Lung, and Blood Institute PTCA Registry. Circulation 67, 1983, pp. 723-730.

Douglas, J. S. , Jr. , Gruentzig, A. R. , King, S. B. III, Hollman, J. , Ischinger, T. , Meier, B. , Craver, J. M. , Jones, E. L. , Waller, J. L. , Bone, D. K. , and Guyton, R. : Percutaneous transluminal coronary angioplasty in patients with prior coronary bypass surgery. J Am Coll Cardiol 2, 1983, pp. 746-754.

Giorgi, L. V. , Hartzler, G. O. , Rutherford, B. D. , and
McConahay, D. R.: Angina following total coronary occlusion—
definitive treatment with percutaneous coronary angioplasty
(Abstr.). J Am Coll Cardiol 1, 1983, p. 656.

Gruntzig, A.: Results from coronary angioplasty and implications for the future. Am Heart J 103, 1982, pp. 779-783.

Gruntzig, A. R. , Senning, A. , and Siegenthaler, W. E.: Nonoperative dilatation of coronary-artery stenosis. Percutaneous
transluminal coronary angioplasty. N Engl J Med 301, 1979,
pp. 61-68.

Health and Public Policy Committee, American College of
Physicians: Percutaneous transluminal angioplasty. Ann Intern
Med 99, 1983, pp. 864-869.

Holmes, D. R. , Vliestra, R. E. , Reeder, G. S. , Bresnaham,
J. F. , Smith, H. C. , Bove, A. A. , and Schaff, H. V.:
Elective percutaneous transluminal coronary angioplasty of
total coronary arterial occlusions not associated with acute
infarction (Abstr.). J Am Coll Cardiol 1, 1983, p. 656.

Jones, E. L. and King, S. B.: Intraoperative angioplasty in
the treatment of coronary artery disease. J Am Coll Cardiol
1, 1983, pp. 970-971.

Kent, K. M. , Bonow, R. O. , Rosing, D. R. , Ewels, C. J. ,
Lipson, L. C. , McIntosh, C. L. , Bacharach, S. , Green, M. ,
and Epstein, S. E.: Improved myocardial function during
exercise after successful percutaneous transluminal coronary
angioplasty. N Engl J Med 306, 1982, pp. 441-446.

Kent, K. M.: Percutaneous transluminal coronary angioplasty.
Past, present, and future. Council in Clinical Cardiology Newsletter (Amer. Heart Assoc.) 7, 1982, pp. 2-8.

Kent, K. M. , Bentivoglio, L. G. , Block, P. C. , Cowley, M. J. ,
Dorros, G. , Gosselin, A. J. , Gruntzig, A. , Myler, R. K. ,
Simpson, J. , Stertzer, S. H. , Williams, D. O. , Fisher, L. ,
Gillespie, M. J. , Detre, K. , Kelsey, S. , Mullin, S. M. , and
Mouk, M. B.: Percutaneous transluminal coronary angioplasty:
Report from the registry of the National Heart, Lung, and Blood
Institute. Am J Cardiol 49, 1982, pp. 2011-2020.

King, S. B. III: Indications for coronary arteriography and coronary angioplasty. Cardiovasc Rev Rep 4, 1983, pp. 625-632.

Meier, B. , Gruentzig, A. R. , King, S. B. III, Douglas, J. R. , Jr. , Hollman, J. , Ischinger, T. , Aueron, F. , and Galan, K. : Risk of side branch occlusion during coronary angioplasty. Am J Cardiol 53, 1984, pp. 10-17.

Meyer, J. , Merx, W. , Schmitz, H. , Erbel, R. , Kiesslich, T. , Dorr, R. , Lambertz, H. , Bethge, C. , Krebs, W. , Bardos, P. , Minale, C. , Messmer, B. J. , and Effert, S. : Percutaneous transluminal coronary angioplasty immediately after intra-coronary streptolysis of transmural myocardial infarction. Circulation 66, 1982, pp. 905-913.

Vliestra, R. E. , Holmes, D. R. , Reeder, G. S. , Jr. , Mock, M. B. , Smith, H. C. , Bove, A. A. , Bresnaham, J. F. , and Pichler, J. M. : Balloon angioplasty in multivessel coronary disease: Mayo Clin Proc 58, 1983, pp. 563-567.

Chapter 11

PRIMARY AND SECONDARY PREVENTION OF ARTERIOSCLEROTIC HEART DISEASE

INTRODUCTION

Over the past 15 years, there has been a steady and dramatic decline in the mortality rate due to ischemic heart disease in this country. To an extent, this has probably resulted from important developments in the diagnosis and treatment of this disease. It appears more likely, however, that the major portion of this declining mortality has been due to reduction in the incidence and progression of ischemic heart disease as a result of preventative measures. The identification of "risk factors" contributing to the development of ischemic heart disease and the increased awareness of these factors by the general population has resulted in successful efforts by the American population to reduce the prevalence and extent of these factors. Several recent landmark studies have clarified some basic questions on the causes and prevention of ischemic heart disease, although major controversies continue to exist in this area. In this chapter, the current knowledge of this subject is reviewed and practical guidelines are given according to contemporary viewpoints.

THE PATHOGENESIS OF ATHEROSCLEROSIS

Although the pathogenesis of atherosclerosis is still not well understood, there is considerable evidence that the primary events consist of a combination of endothelial damage and proliferation of smooth muscle cells in the arterial wall. This damage is largely caused by circulating cholesterol (and more specifically by the low-density lipoprotein which is the major carrier of circulating cholesterol) with subsequent attachment of mononuclear cells to the endothelium which then migrate into the endothelial cells. This is accompanied by platelet deposition and disintegration with the release of a platelet component (platelet-derived growth factor) which promotes smooth muscle cell proliferation in the arterial wall. Additional endothelial injury, which may result from hypertension, smoking, or other factors, seems to accelerate the athero- sclerotic process. In experimental animal models, accelerated atherosclerosis can be produced with atherogenic diets (very high cholesterol and saturated fat content) with or without associated direct arterial wall injury. Experimental athero- sclerosis can be prevented in animals with the use of drugs which lower serum cholesterol. Recent studies have also demonstrated that these lesions can be inhibited by substances that block the entry of calcium into the arterial wall and also by interferon inducers.

Up until very recently, there was only indirect evidence in humans that atherosclerosis could be prevented or retarded, but there is now evidence that reduction in serum cholesterol does reduce the incidence of mortality and morbidity in athero- sclerotic cardiovascular disease. The prevention of athero- sclerotic plaques and of subsequent symptomatic cardiovascular disease is known as "primary prevention" of ischemic heart disease. "Secondary prevention" refers to prevention of further manifestations of ischemic heart disease once the disease has already become clinically manifest. Ideally, this should be accomplished by means of regression of atherosclerotic plaques. Such plaque regression has, in fact, been demonstrated in hyper- cholesterolemic patients with peripheral atherosclerosis who have been treated with drugs to lower their serum cholesterol. Similar results have not been reproduced in coronary artery disease, where spontaneous or induced regression of plaques is distinctly unusual. However, an important recent study has demonstrated that the progression of coronary atherosclerosis can be retarded by reduction of serum cholesterol in hyper- cholesterolemic patients.

RISK FACTORS AND THEIR MODIFICATION

Both the primary and secondary prevention of ischemic heart disease have been based upon the principle of risk factor modifi- cation. Multiple epidemiologic studies have demonstrated that the presence of certain risk factors is associated with an in- creased incidence of ischemic heart disease, especially in younger persons. Although not all persons who develop ischemic heart disease have one or more such risk factors, the likelihood of development of ischemic heart disease is increased by the number of risk factors present in the given individual or given population. Certain risk factors such as age, sex, and family history are nonmodifiable, whereas others are modifiable to varying extents (Table 11-1). The role of risk factor modification

Table 11-1.   Risk Factors

I. NONMODIFIABLE
   A.   Age
   B.   Sex
   C.   Race
   D.   Family history

II. PARTIALLY MODIFIABLE
   A.   Hyperlipidemia
   B.   Hypertension
   C.   Diabetes mellitus
   D.   Obesity
   E.   Personality
   F.   Geographic area
   G.   Hardness of drinking water

III. TOTALLY MODIFIABLE
   A.   Smoking
   B.   Physical activity
   C.   Oral contraceptives
   D.   Coffee and **caffeine**

---

in the primary and secondary prevention of ischemic heart disease is a highly controversial subject, with facts gradually emerging from multiple completed and ongoing studies. The following is a summary of the role of each known risk factor in the development of ischemic heart disease, and where applicable, the evidence of the role of modification of these factors in the prevention of ischemic disease.

NONMODIFIABLE RISK FACTORS

1. Age

Both the incidence and mortality of ischemic heart disease increases directly with increasing age in both males and females.

2. Sex

The prevalence of ischemic heart disease is significantly higher in males than in females of the same age, and the risk is much higher in females of the same age who are postmenopausal compared to females who are still menstruating.

3. Race

Prior to 1968 Caucasians in the United States had a higher age-adjusted death rate from ischemic heart disease than non-Caucasians, but since then, the ratio has reversed (up to the age of 65). There are also differences in mortality rates in ischemic heart disease between other ethnic groups living in the same country, which cannot be explained by environmental factors and appear to be due to racial factors.

4. Family History

There is a very high association between family history of atherosclerotic heart disease and subsequent development of this disease in offspring or siblings. To a large extent, this appears to be due to the hereditary aspects of other known risk factors including hypercholesterolemia, diabetes mellitus, and hypertension, but there also appears to be some independent genetic factors as well.

PARTIALLY MODIFIABLE RISK FACTORS

1. Hyperlipidemia (hypercholesterolemia)

Evidence has been progressively mounting to implicate the role of hypercholesterolemia in the development of atherosclerotic coronary artery disease. The evidence is now very strong that there is a direct relationship between serum cholesterol level and the risk of coronary artery disease. The majority of cholesterol in the blood is synthesized in the liver and is predominantly transported in the blood in the form of low-density lipoprotein (LDL). A small percentage of the total amount of cholesterol in the blood exists in the form of high-density lipoprotein (HDL), with an even smaller percentage in the form of very low-density lipoprotein (VLDL). It appears that the lipid fraction most directly associated with atherosclerosis is the LDL fraction, the serum concentration of which correlates best with the risk of coronary artery disease. In contrast, there is a reverse relationship between the serum HDL level and the risk of coronary artery disease, in that the higher the HDL, the lower the risk of coronary artery disease. The prevalence of coronary artery disease is twice as high in persons with an HDL level at 30 mg/dl compared to persons with an HDL level of 60 mg/dl. Furthermore, the serum LDL/HDL ratio is an even better indicator than either the HDL or LDL alone in risk prediction. Men with an LDL/HDL ratio of 3.55 have an average risk ratio of coronary heart disease, while a ratio of 1.0 is associated with one-half the average risk, and a ratio of 8.0 is associated with three times the average risk. HDL particles themselves are composed of approximately 50% lipid (1/3 of which is cholesterol) and approximately 50% apolipoprotein. The major apolipoprotein is termed apolipoprotein A-I, which can now be measured chemically, and appears to be an even more specific and sensitive indicator of the likelihood of coronary artery disease than is the level of HDL, according to recent studies. The apparent explanation for the inverse relationship between HDL level and coronary artery disease risk is that the HDL in the serum acts to transport cholesterol from the peripheral tissues (including the arterial wall) to the liver, where it is excreted via the bile acid excretory pathway. Whereas total cholesterol level and LDL cholesterol are influenced by diet as well as by hereditary factors, HDL level is influenced only slightly by diet but is influenced by a number of other factors: HDL can be increased by exercise, moderate alcohol intake, and weight reduction, while it is decreased by smoking, obesity, poorly controlled diabetes mellitus, and progesterone-containing oral contraceptives.

Although there is still considerable debate over the relationship of serum triglycerides to coronary atherosclerosis, it now appears that serum triglyceride level is not an important independent factor in the risk of atherosclerotic heart disease. Measurement of the serum triglyceride level is useful, however, for the calculation of LDL level (LDL = Total cholesterol - [HDL + Triglyceride/5]) and as an indicator for the presence of a lipid disorder.

2. Hypertension

Both systolic and diastolic hypertension are clearly associated with increased morbidity and mortality due to coronary artery disease, and the level of hypertension is directly proportionate to the risk. There is increasing evidence that treatment of all levels of hypertension will decrease the risk of mortality and morbidity of this disease.

3. Diabetes Mellitus

There is a significant increase in the incidence of ischemic heart disease in persons with diabetes mellitus compared to non-diabetics and this appears to be independent of other risk factors. Treatment of diabetes with insulin does not seem to reduce the subsequent risk of ischemic heart disease, and treatment with

certain oral hypoglycemic agents may actually increase the
risk of coronary heart disease.

4. Obesity

Although the association between obesity and coronary artery
disease has long been recognized, it has only recently been
demonstrated that obesity is a significant independent predictor
of coronary artery disease risk, especially in females.

5. Personality

The risk of coronary artery disease has been associated with
personality type, in that the "type A" personality, described as
compulsive, competitive, ambitious, impatient, and aggressive
is "coronary prone," having twice the risk of coronary disease
as does the "type B" personality type, who is relaxed and easy-
going. To a small extent, personality type is modifiable, but
the result of such modification on subsequent development or
progression of coronary heart disease is unknown.

6. Geographic Area

There are marked variations of incidence and in mortality of
ischemic heart disease both within a given country and between
countries. There are multiple possible explanations for these
differences, such as race, diet, and climate, but it is largely
unexplained. One additional factor which may play a role is the
hardness of drinking water, in that those areas with "soft"
water have a higher incidence of coronary heart disease than in
areas with "hard" water.

TOTALLY MODIFIABLE RISK FACTORS

1. Smoking

Cigarette smoking is clearly a strong independent risk factor
for the development of coronary artery disease, especially
in younger men. There is a direct relationship between the
number of cigarettes smoked and the risk of coronary artery
disease, but no apparent relationship between either the tar and
nicotine content of cigarettes or filtered vs nonfiltered cigarettes
and incidence of ischemic heart disease. Most important, it
has been demonstrated that reduction or cessation of smoking
is associated with a marked decrease in subsequent risk as well
as mortality from coronary artery disease. This applies both
to the primary and secondary prevention of ischemic heart
disease.

2. Physical Activity

The relationship between physical activity and the incidence of
coronary heart disease has been controversial. Several epi-
demiological studies have shown that persons engaging in regular
physical activity have a lower incidence of coronary artery disease compared to sedentary persons, although other studies
have not consistently demonstrated this relationship. The
positive relationship between exercise and HDL levels may be
a factor in protection from coronary artery disease, but this is
yet to be established. A recent experimental study in monkeys
demonstrated a protective effect of moderate physical conditioning in the development of coronary artery disease, but this protective effect has not yet been demonstrated in humans.

3. Oral Contraceptives

The use of oral contraceptives is associated with increased risk
of cardiovascular disease, including myocardial infarction,
especially in females over age 35 who are heavy smokers or
have other risk factors. The possible mechanisms whereby
oral contraceptives result in increased risk include increased
thrombogenicity as well as accelerated atherogenesis due to
increased blood pressure, decreased glucose tolerance, and
decreased HDL levels.

4. Coffee and Caffeine

The role of coffee and caffeine in increasing the risk of coronary
artery disease has also been a somewhat controversial subject,
but as of the present time, there seems to be little direct relationship between coffee and caffeine in cardiovascular risk.

MULTIPLE RISK FACTORS

Each of the major risk factors is a variable in regard to the
degree of risk of development of coronary artery disease, such
that the degree of risk increases directly with the level of
serum cholesterol (or LDL) (or inversely with the level of
HDL), and directly with the number of cigarettes smoked and
with the degree of hypertension, as well as with increasing
age. By combining the degree of risk from each risk factor
present, an overall assessment can be made of the risk of
coronary heart disease in an individual. Obviously, the
higher number of risk factors present as well as the higher
the degree of abnormality of each risk factor, the higher the

individual risk. The Handbook of Coronary Risk Probability,
published by the American Heart Association and based on
data obtained from the Framingham study, gives an estimate
of risk development of coronary heart disease over a 6-year
period in asymptomatic individuals without known coronary
heart disease based on values of serum cholesterol, blood
pressure, and for presence or absence of carbohydrate intolerance, left ventricular hypertrophy on the electrocardiogram,
and cigarette smoking. For example, a 40-year-old man who
is a nonsmoker, has a systolic blood pressure of 105 mmHg,
a serum cholesterol of 185 mg/dl, and no LVH on ECG has a
0.7% likelihood of developing symptomatic coronary heart
disease in 6 years, while a man the same age who smokes,
has glucose intolerance, a systolic blood pressure of 180 mmHg,
a serum cholesterol of 310 mg/dl, and LVH present on the
ECG has a 26.6% chance of developing symptomatic coronary
heart disease in the same time period, or 39 times the risk!
More recent risk tables include LDL and HDL cholesterol
as well as LDL/HDL ratio rather than total serum cholesterol,
and provide an even better estimate of risk.

PRIMARY PREVENTION OF
CORONARY HEART DISEASE

The prevention of coronary heart disease has long been and
continues to be one of the most important public health goals
in this country. To what extent this is achievable has been a
very controversial issue, with opinions ranging from the concept that coronary heart disease is not a preventable disease
to the concept that as much as a two-thirds reduction in cardiovascular disease mortality in this country is possible by a
slight reduction in serum cholesterol and blood pressure and
by elimination of cigarette smoking. Most authorities now feel
that even if coronary heart disease cannot be prevented, at
least some significant impact can be made on reducing cardiovascular mortality and morbidity by modification of risk
factors. There is at least indirect evidence that a large part
of the recent reduction in mortality from coronary heart disease
in this country is due directly to individual voluntary risk factor
modification. Certain risk factors such as age, sex, and family history cannot be modified at all; some can be totally reversed, such as smoking, obesity, sedentary life-style, and
the use of oral contraceptives; and others including serum
cholesterol (both LDL and HDL), blood pressure, and glucose
intolerance and personality can be modified to a variable extent.
It has been well demonstrated that cessation of smoking and

correction of hypertension is associated with reduced risk of coronary heart disease as well as reduced risk of noncardiovascular conditions. Although correction of obesity and glucose intolerance has not been demonstrated as of yet to affect cardiovascular morbidity and mortality, little argument can be made against modification of these risk factors for general health reasons. Oral contraceptives can be discontinued or modified, and the current oral contraceptives contain lower concentrations of estrogen and progesterone, which has resulted in a reduction of cardiovascular risk from the use of these agents.

The area of greatest controversy and potentially greatest impact is the role of modification of serum cholesterol in the prevention of coronary heart disease. There is considerable evidence that the level of serum cholesterol (and especially LDL) correlates directly with the risk of development of coronary heart disease and also that the amount of cholesterol and saturated fats in the diet affects (to a variable extent within individuals) the serum cholesterol and LDL cholesterol levels. The two areas of greatest controversy involve the questions: (1) To what extent will reduction of serum cholesterol prevent (or reverse) coronary heart disease? and (2) To what extent will modification of diet prevent (or reverse) coronary heart disease? There is little disagreement that in familial hyperlipoproteinemia, in which serum cholesterol is greatly elevated, the incidence of premature arteriosclerosis is very high, and that this condition should be treated aggressively to decrease this risk. In individuals with "normal" cholesterol values, however, it is unclear to what extent reduction in serum cholesterol by diet will affect subsequent development of coronary heart disease. Although "normal" serum cholesterol in adults has been reported to be up to 260 mg/dl, this value is derived from the healthy adult U. S. population, and this figure does not imply that serum cholesterol levels up to 260 mg/dl are ideal. There appears to be a "threshold" of serum cholesterol in the risk of arteriosclerosis in that any value of serum cholesterol of less than 200 mg/dl is associated with a low risk of coronary disease, whereas values greater than 200 mg/dl are associated with progressive increase in risk. A serum cholesterol of over 268 mg/dl is associated with twice the risk for cardiovascular disease compared to a cholesterol of under 218 mg/dl. Several studies have now shown that reduction in serum cholesterol by a diet low in saturated fat and low in cholesterol can result in a reduced incidence of myocardial infarction and reduced mortality from coronary heart disease. In the recent and much publicized multiple risk factor intervention trial (MRFIT) "high-risk" men were assigned to either a special intervention program

to treat hypertension, discourage smoking, and lower serum
cholesterol with dietary means, or to a group in which no special
counseling in these areas was given. The results of this study
were recently reported and somewhat surprisingly showed no
significant difference in mortality from coronary heart disease
between the special intervention and the control groups. While
a number of possible explanations were considered, at least
one of the reasons appeared to be due to a significant reduction
in risk factors by the control group as well as by the special
intervention group. Another study from Oslo, Norway was more
positive, showing a 47% reduction in myocardial infarction and
sudden death in the group treated with diet and antismoking
advice.

The most important and convincing study on the primary
prevention of coronary artery disease by cholesterol reduction
was just recently reported. The Lipid Research Clinics Program Primary Prevention Trial Results showed conclusively
that reduction of total serum cholesterol (by an average of
13.4%) and LDL cholesterol (by an average of 20.3%) in individuals with familial hypercholesterolemia (serum cholesterol of
265 mg/dl or greater) with diet and cholestyramine (a cholesterol-lowering drug) resulted in a 19% reduction in coronary
risk (24% reduction in death due to coronary disease and 19%
reduction of nonfatal myocardial infarction) in an average
followup of 7-1/2 years. Equally important, there was a 20-25%
reduction in new positive exercise tests, new onset of angina,
and need for coronary artery bypass surgery in the treated
group. Moreover, there was a direct relationship between the
extent of cholesterol reduction and the degree of risk reduction,
so that for every 1% fall in cholesterol there was a 2% reduction in the incidence of coronary disease. In the patients who took
the full dose of cholestyramine (24 g/day), there was a 25% fall
in total cholesterol and a 35% fall in LDL level, with a resultant
49% reduction in the incidence of coronary disease!

Based on the evidence that dietary control of serum cholesterol can have a significant impact on the development of coronary heart disease, a major controversy still exists whether
all persons in this country should try to modify their diet to
lower their serum cholesterol or whether only persons at
higher risk because of elevated serum cholesterol should modify
their diet. The Food and Nutrition Board of the National
Academy of Sciences recently stated that persons with no
apparent hypercholesterolemia should not limit their intake of
dietary cholesterol, since they are not at increased risk for
development of coronary heart disease due to this factor.
Supporting this approach is the fact that 40-50% of the American

population have a normal serum cholesterol (<200 mg/dl) and would not significantly decrease their risk of coronary heart disease by the unnecessary restrictions in diet. The American Heart Association, however, takes an opposing stand and feels that general modifications of the American diet are necessary in order to make a significant impact on coronary heart disease in this country. They currently recommend the following modifications of diet:

1. Reduce the proportionate calories derived from fats from the current average of 40% to 30%.
2. Saturated fats should make up no more than 10% of daily caloric intake.
3. Unsaturated fats should account for about (but not more than) 10% of daily caloric intake.
4. Carbohydrates should supply 55% of daily calories (an increase from the current average of 45%).
5. Cholesterol intake should be reduced to less than 300 mg per day.

The American Heart Association also recently made dietary recommendations for children over two years of age:

1. Total fat intake should be approximately 30% of calories, with 10% or less from saturated fat, approximately 10% from monosaturated fat, and less than 10% from polyunsaturated fat.
2. Daily cholesterol intake should be approximately 100 mg of cholesterol per 1,000 calories, not to exceed a total of 300 mg per day.
3. Carbohydrate intake should account for 55% of calories.

An alternate approach to the modification of diet of the entire population, is to do blood lipid screening of all persons felt to have increased risk of coronary heart disease (because of the presence of risk factors other than hyperlipidemia). A cholesterol, HDL level, and fasting triglyceride level should be obtained for such persons, from which LDL cholesterol can be calculated according to the formula: LDL = Total cholesterol - (HDL + triglycerides/5). By measuring serum lipids, patients can be separated into high-, average-, and low-risk groups for coronary heart disease on the basis of this one risk factor, and diet can be individualized according to lipid level. Persons with a total serum cholesterol of less than 200 mg/dl do not need any special diet or other treatment to lower serum cholesterol. Persons with a total cholesterol of 200 to 240 mg/dl should have at least one repeat determination made at another time. If the value is still in the same range, an HDL and triglyceride determination should be made and LDL/HDL ratio should be calculated. If the ratio is greater than 3:1, such persons should have dietary instruction for lowering serum cholesterol, especially if they are under the age of 50. Persons with cholesterol levels between 240 and 265 should also have serum HDL and triglyceride levels determined and should also have dietary reduction of cholesterol following the same guidelines, especially if under age 65. In persons over this age, it is unclear to what extent reduction in serum cholesterol levels will reduce the risk of coronary disease. Persons with cholesterol levels over 265 mg/dl should have secondary causes for hypercholesterolemia looked for (diabetes, obesity, or liver or renal disease) and the secondary causes should be corrected if possible. If no secondary cause is found, dietary instruction should be given and repeat lipid determinations made in 3 months. If no significant reduction occurs despite adherence to diet, pharmacological therapy is indicated (see below). Patients with serum cholesterol values in this range frequently have familial hyperlipoproteinemia, in which there is a genetic defect in lipid metabolism, and these persons need pharmacologic therapy, since dietary management alone is ineffective, and these patients have accelerated atherosclerosis.

DIETARY TREATMENT OF
HYPERCHOLESTEROLEMIA

The American Heart Association has recently recommended a stepwise dietary program for the treatment of hypercholesterolemia. Phase I is the same diet recommended for the general public, while phases II and III are progressive reductions in fat and cholesterol which are prescribed as necessary to bring the serum cholesterol into recommended range:

| | % of Total Calories as: | | | |
	Fat	Carbohydrate	Protein	Total Cholesterol (mg/day)
Phase I	30	55	15	300
Phase II	25	60	15	200-250
Phase III	20	65	15	100-150

PHARMACOLOGIC TREATMENT OF
HYPERLIPIDEMIA

Pharmacologic therapy (Table 11-2) is usually initiated with a
bile sequestering agent, which increases the excretion of
cholesterol in the stool and results in a 15-30% decrease in
serum cholesterol and LDL cholesterol without a significant
effect on HDL level.   The two available bile sequestering
agents are cholestyramine (Questran) and colestipol (Colestid).
Another drug which increases the excretion of cholesterol in
the stool is D-thyroxine (Choloxin), but the side effects of this
drug limit its usefulness.   Nicotinic acid (niacin) is another
effective drug in lowering cholesterol and LDL and works indirectly by decreasing synthesis of VLDL.   It must be given
in high doses and usually in conjunction with bile sequestering
agents to lower serum cholesterol, and is also associated with
significant side effects, but does have the advantage of increasing
HDL levels as well.   When combined with colestipol, as much as
a 40% decrease in serum cholesterol and a 50% decrease in LDL
level has been reported, with a 32% increase in HDL.

Probucol (Lorelco) is also an effective drug for lowering
serum cholesterol and LDL levels with the unfortunate effect
of also lowering serum HDL levels.   When combined with
colestipol, probucol results in an average reduction of 30% in
total and LDL-cholesterol, with no change in the LDL:HDL
ratio and results in minimal side effects.   Gemfibrozil (Lopid)
is a new drug that lowers triglyceride more than cholesterol
but does have a significant effect on lowering both cholesterol
and LDL levels and increasing HDL levels and may turn out
to be an important drug in the treatment of hypercholesterolemia.

Another new and very promising drug for lowering serum
cholesterol is compactin, which inhibits cholesterol synthesis
and stimulates the production of LDL receptors in the liver,
thus lowering serum LDL levels without affecting HDL levels.
Mevolin is an analog of compactin, with even more potent
cholesterol-lowering effect.   When combined with cholestyramine
or colestipol, compactin or mevolin is an extremely effective
combination resulting in a 40-45% reduction in serum cholesterol
and 53% reduction in LDL level. At the present time, however,
neither compactin nor mevolin are FDA approved or available
clinically.   Another agent, Beta-sitosterol (Cytellin), inhibits
cholesterol absorption and results in a modest decrease in
cholesterol but appears to be counteracted by a compensatory
increase in cholesterol synthesis.

Clofibrate (Atromid-S) is a commonly used drug for hyperlipidemia, but it affects VLDL levels predominantly, with only

Table 11-2. Comparative Effects of Clinically Available Drugs for Hypercholesterolemia

Generic Name	Trade Name	Maintenance Dose (Daily)	Effect on Total Cholesterol	Effect on HDL Cholesterol	Principle Side Effects
Cholestyramine	Questran, Cuemid	12–32 g	↓15–30%	Slight↑	Abdominal discomfort, constipation or diarrhea
Colestipol	Colestid	15–30 g	↓15–30%	Slight↑	Same as cholestyramine
Nicotinic acid (Niacin)	—	2–8 g	↓20–30%	Slight↑	Flushing, nausea, diarrhea, pruritis
D-Thyroxine	Choloxin	2–8 g	↓15–20%	—	Arrhythmias, angina
Probucol	Lorelco	1 g	↓18–22%	—	Diarrhea, nausea
Gemfibrozil	Lopid	800–120 mg	↓10–16%	17–25%↑	Nausea, epigastric pain, diarrhea
Clofibrate	Atromid-S	1–2 g	↓10–12%	—	Nausea, diarrhea, cholelithiasis

a slight decrease in cholesterol level and is probably not indicated in the treatment of hypercholesterolemia, except when
associated with type III hyperlipoproteinemia (broad-beta disease), which is relatively rare and is characterized by increased
cholesterol and triglyceride and is diagnosed by lipoprotein
electrophoresis.

OTHER MEASURES FOR PRIMARY PREVENTION

Another approach, which has been applied more to secondary
prevention than to primary prevention thus far, involves interfering with the action of platelets in arteriosclerosis. It is felt
that platelets are involved in arteriosclerosis in several ways:
when endothelial injury occurs (perhaps as a result of LDL induced damage), platelet aggregation occurs at the site, forming
microthrombin, which contributes to plaque formation. As a
result of platelet aggregation, thromboxane A_2 is released by
platelets, which not only causes more platelet aggregation but
also results in localized arterial vasospasm. Perhaps of
greatest importance, the platelets also release another factor,
"platelet-derived growth factor," which leads to proliferation of
arterial small muscle cells, which result in plaque formation.
Aspirin blocks the formation of thromboxane A_2, which is the
mechanism responsible for its inhibition of blood clotting.
(High-dose aspirin also blocks the formation of prostacyclin,
which is produced by the arterial endothelial cells and counter-
acts the actions of thromboxane A_2.) The use of low-dose
aspirin in secondary prevention has already been commented
upon in Chapter 8 and will be discussed further below. This
approach is now also being looked at in primary prevention,
and a large prospective American study is now underway to test
this. In addition, a number of other drugs are also being in-
vestigated which either inhibit thromboxane A_2 or stimulate
the formation of prostacyclin.

Another approach involves the use of substances derived
from fish oils (eicosapentaenoic acid [EPA] and docosa-
hexaenoic acid [DHA]), which act by both inhibiting the formation of thromboxane A_2 and also by decreasing plasma cholesterol
and triglyceride. Consumption of cold-water oily fish (mackerel,
salmon, and sardines) accomplishes the same result as taking
these substances and apparently accounts for the reduced incidence of atherosclerosis in populations that consume such
fish in large quantities.

Still a different approach in the primary prevention of arteriosclerosis involves the concept that the arteriosclerotic process
also involves calcium entry into the arterial wall. Drugs that

inhibit excess deposition of calcium in the arterial wall, such as lanthanum and diphosphonates, have recently been shown to inhibit plaque formation in experimental animals and may turn out to be useful in primary prevention in humans. Calcium antagonists and chelating agents might also be effective. Still another experimental approach that appears to have promise involves the administration of interferon inducers, which inhibit smooth muscle cell proliferation and appear to inhibit the development of arteriosclerosis.

SECONDARY PREVENTION OF
CORONARY HEART DISEASE

The goal of secondary prevention is to slow the progression and perhaps even reverse some of the arteriosclerotic process which has become clinically manifest (as angina pectoris, myocardial infarction, or asymptomatic but clinically detectable coronary artery disease). In the most limited sense, it refers to a decrease in the incidence of subsequent clinical cardiac events in patients with known coronary heart disease. Although regression of an arteriosclerosis has been demonstrated in experimental animals by means of marked reduction in serum cholesterol as well as by exercise training, regression of arteriosclerosis in humans has not been demonstrated to occur with any known intervention as of the present time. Thus far, with the exception of cessation of cigarette smoking, modification of other risk factors, including hypercholesterolemia, hypertension, diabetes mellitus, and obesity, has not yet been demonstrated to lessen the subsequent incidence of cardiac events or cardiac mortality in patients with established coronary artery disease.

Recently, however, a decreased progression of angiographically demonstrated coronary disease has been demonstrated with the use of either cholestyramine or colestipol. In the recently reported results of the NHLBI Type II Coronary Intervention Study, only 12% of patients with significant coronary artery lesions and type II hypercholesterolemia treated with cholestyramine plus diet showed progression of disease over 5 years compared to 33% of patients treated with placebo and diet. Moreover, there was an inverse relationship between progression of disease and increase in HDL and decrease in LDL-cholesterol. The best predictors of progression were changes in HDL/Total cholesterol and HDL/LDL-cholesterol ratios. Similar results were found in another study using colestipol rather than cholestyramine to reduce serum cholesterol.

The use of platelet-inhibiting drugs (aspirin, dipyridamole, or sulfinpyrazone) following acute myocardial infarction has been shown to have a trend toward reducing subsequent acute myocardial infarction and mortality, although the results have thus far not been conclusive and the effective doses have not been established. In the absence of contraindications, the routine use of aspirin at a dose of 325 mg every 2 to 4 days may be justified following acute myocardial infarction. The use of low-dose aspirin also appears to be very effective in secondary prevention in the course of unstable angina pectoris. The routine use of a beta-blocking drug following acute myocardial infarction has been shown to reduce subsequent mortality and reinfarction rates if the drug is started soon after the initial myocardial infarction and there are no contraindications. Several beta-blocking drugs have been found effective for this use, with little difference between the results with different drugs and different dosages. The duration of protection with this therapy is not known, but it appears to be at least 3 years.

Although major controversies exist in the areas of primary and secondary prevention of arteriosclerotic heart disease, it is clear that a great deal has been learned in recent years, and that the goal of prevention is now feasible.

REFERENCES

PATHOGENESIS OF ATHEROSCLEROSIS

Bukley, B. H. : Pathophysiology of coronary heart disease, in McIntosh, H. D. (Ed.), "Baylor College of Medicine Cardiology Series," Vol. 6, No. 2, 1983, pp. 5-27.

Kuo, P. T. : Lipoproteins, platelets, and prostaglandins in atherosclerosis. Am Heart J 102, 1981, pp. 949-953.

Majno, G. , Zand, T. , Nunnari, J. J. , and Joris, I. : The diet/atherosclerosis connection: new insights. J Cardiovasc Med 9, 1984, pp. 21-30.

Niewiarowski, S. and Rao, K. : Contribution of thrombogenic factors to the pathogenesis of atherosclerosis. Prog Cardiovasc Dis 26, 1983, pp. 197-222.

Ross, R. : Factors influencing atherogenesis, in Hurst, J. W. (Ed.), "The Heart," 5th Edition, McGraw-Hill, New York, 1982, pp. 935-958.

Wissler, R. W. : Principles of the pathogenesis of athero-sclerosis, in Braunwald, E. (Ed.), "Heart Disease," 2nd Edition, W. B. Saunders, Philadelphia, 1984, pp. 1183-1204.

RISK FACTORS AND ATHEROSCLEROSIS (GENERAL)

AHA Committee Report: Risk factors and coronary disease.
A statement for physicians. Circulation 62, 1980, pp. 449A-
455A.

Castelli, W. P.: Epidemiology of coronary heart disease: the
Framingham study. Am J Med 76, 2/27/84, pp. 4-12.

Gordon, T. and Kannel, W. B.: Multiple risk factors for
predicting coronary heart disease: The concept, accuracy,
and application. Am Heart J 103, 1982, pp. 1031-1039.

Kannel, W. B.: Handbook of Coronary Risk Probability.
American Heart Association, 1972.

Kannel, W. B. and Schatzkin, A.: Risk factor analysis. Prog
Cardiovasc Dis 26, 1984, pp. 309-332.

Levy, R. I. and Feinleib, M.: Risk factors for coronary artery
disease and their management, in Braunwald, E. (Ed.), "Heart
Disease," 2nd Edition, W. B. Saunders, Philadelphia, 1984,
pp. 1205-1234.

Vliestra, R. E., Frye, R. L., Kronmal, R. A., Sim, D. A.,
Tristani, F. E., Killip, T., III, and participants in the Coronary Artery Surgery Study: Risk factors and angiographic
coronary artery disease: A report from the coronary artery
surgery study (CASS). Circulation 62, 1980, pp. 254-261.

DIET, LIPIDS, AND ATHEROSCLEROSIS

AHA Committee Report: Rationale of the diet-heart statement
of the American Heart Association. Circulation 65, 1982, pp.
839A-854A.

AHA Committee Report: Diet in the healthy child. Circulation
67, 1983, pp. 1711-1714.

American Heart Association: Diet and coronary heart disease.
1978, pp. 1-6.

Consensus Conference, Office of Medical Application of Research, National Institutes of Health: Treatment of hyper-
triglyceridemia. JAMA 251, 1984, pp. 1196-1200.

Council on Scientific Affairs: Dietary and pharmacologic
therapy for the lipid risk factors. JAMA 250, 1983, pp.
1873-1879.

Dujovne, C. A. , Krehbiel, P. , Decoursey, S. , Jackson, B. ,
Chernoff, S. B. , Pitterman, A. , and Garty, M. : Probucol
with colestipol in the treatment of hypercholesterolemia.
Ann Intern Med 100, 1984, pp. 477-482.

Ehnholm, G. , Huttunen, J. K. , Pietinen, P. , Leino, U. ,
Mutanen, M. , Kostiainen, E. , Pikkarainen, T. , Dougherty, R. ,
Iacono, J. , and Puska, P. : Effect of serum lipoproteins in a
population with a high risk of coronary heart disease. New
Engl J Med 307, 1982, pp. 850-855.

Glueck, C. J. : Colestipol and probucol: Treatment of primary
and familial hypercholesterolemia and amelioration of atherosclerosis. Ann Intern Med 96, 1982, pp. 475-482.

Glueck, C. J. : Relationships of lipid disorders to coronary
heart disease. Am J Med 74, 5/23/83, pp. 10-14.

Gotto, A. M. , Jr. (Ed.): Symposium on high-density lipoprotein and coronary artery disease: Effects of diet, exercise,
and pharmacologic intervention. Am J Cardiol 52, 1983, pp.
1B-43B.

Gordon, T. , Kannel, W. R. , Castelli, W. P. , and Dawber,
T. R. : Lipoproteins, cardiovascular disease and death. The
Framingham study. Arch Intern Med 141, 1981, pp. 1128-1131.

Grundy, S. M. : Future trends in the prevention of coronary
heart disease. Part I. Can dietary change prevent coronary
heart disease? in Yu, P. N. , and Goodwin, T. F. (Eds.),
"Progress in Cardiology," Vol. 10, Lea & Febiger, Philadelphia, 1981, pp. 13-21.

Havel, R. T. : Experience with individual lipid-lowering drugs:
Nicotinic acid. Cardiovasc Rev Rep 3, 1982, pp. 1187-1197.

HunningLake, D. B. : Pharmacologic therapy for the hyper-
lipidemic patient. Am J Med 74, 5/23/83, pp. 19-22.

Illingworth, D. R. , Rapp, T. H. , Phillipson, B. E. , and
Connor, W. E. : Colestipol plus nicotinic acid in treatment of
heterozygous familial hypercholesterolemia. Lancet 1, 1981,
pp. 296-297.

Kriesberg, A. : Lipids, lipoproteins, apolipoproteins, and atherosclerosis. (Editorial). Ann Intern Med 99, 1983, pp. 713-715.

Kuo, P. T. : Hyperlipoproteinemia and atherosclerosis: dietary intervention. Am J Med 74, 5/23/83, pp. 15-18.

Lees, R. S. and Lees, A. M. : High-density lipoproteins and the risk of atherosclerosis. New Engl J Med 306, 1982, pp. 1546-1547.

Levy, R. I. : The mechanisms of action of lipid-lowering drugs. Cardiovasc Rev Rep 3, pp. 1167-1172.

Levy, R. I. : Consideration of cholesterol and noncardiovascular mortality. Am Heart J 104, 1982, pp. 327-328.

Levy, R. I. : Current status of the cholesterol controversy. Am J Med 5/23/83, pp. 1-4.

Mabuchi, H. , Sakai, T. , Sakai, Y. , Yoshimura, A. , Watanabe, A. , Wakasugi, T. , Koizumi, T. , and Takeda, R. : Reduction of serum cholesterol in heterozygous patients with familial hyper-cholesterolemia: additive effects of compactin and cholestyra-mine. New Engl J Med 308, 1983, pp. 609-613.

Maciejko, T. T. , Holmes, D. R. , Kottke, B. A. , Zinsmeister, A. R. , Dinh, D. M. , and Mao, S. J. T. : Apolipoprotein A-1 as a marker of angiographically assessed coronary artery dis-ease. New Engl J Med 309, 1983, pp. 385-389.

McNamara, D. J. : Diet and hyperlipodemia. A justifiable debate. Arch Intern Med 192, 1982, pp. 1121-1124.

Medical Letter: Fish oil prevention of atherosclerosis. 24, 1982, pp. 99-100.

Peabody, H. D. : Clinical investigation of gemfibrozil: The treatment of primary hyperlipoproteinemia. Cardiovasc Rev Rep 3, 1982, pp. 1195-1200.

Probstfield, J. L. and Gotto, A. M. : Lipoproteins in health and disease: Diagnosis and management, in McIntosh, H. D. (Ed.), "Baylor College of Medicine Cardiology Series," Vol. 5, 1982, pp. 6-31.

Rifkind, B. M. and Segal, P. : Lipid Research Clinics Program reference values for hyperlipidemia and hypolipidemia. JAMA 250, 1983, pp. 1869-1872.

Samuel, P. : Effects of gemfibrozil on serum lipids. Am J Med 74, 5/23/83, pp. 23-27.

Shekelle, R. S. , Shryock, A. M. , Paul, O. , Lepper, M. , Stamler, J. , Liu, S. , and Raynor, W. J. Jr. : Diet, serum cholesterol and death from coronary heart disease: The Western Electric study. New Engl J Med 304, 1981, pp. 65-70.

Tyroler, H. A. (Ed.): Epidemiology of plasma high-density lipoprotein cholesterol levels. Circulation 62, 1980, pp. IV-1-IV-136.

OTHER RISK FACTORS AND ATHEROSCLEROSIS

Bruce, R. A. : Primary intervention against coronary atherosclerosis by exercise conditioning? New Engl J Med 305, 1981, pp. 1525-1526.

Chobanian, A. V. : The influence of hypertension and other hemodynamic factors in atherogenesis. Prog Cardiovasc Dis 26, 1983, pp. 177-196.

Dalen, J. E. and Hickler, R. B. : Oral contraceptives and cardiovascular disease. Am Heart J 101, 1981, pp. 626-638.

Froelicher, V. F. and Brown, P. : Exercise and coronary heart disease. J Card Rehab 1, 1981, pp. 277-288.

Hamby, R. I. : Hereditary aspects of coronary artery disease. Am Heart J 101, 1981, pp. 639-649.

Harlan, W. R. , Sharrett, A. R. , Weill, H. , Turino, G. M. , Borhani, N. O., and Reshekov, L. : Impact of environment on cardiovascular disease; report of the American Heart Association Task Force on Cardiovascular Disease. Circulation 63, 1981, pp. 242A-271A.

Hubert, H. B. , Feinleib, M. , McNamara, P. M. , and Castelli, W. P. : Obesity as an independent risk factor for cardiovascular disease: A 26 year follow-up of participants in the Framingham study. Circulation 67, 1983, pp. 968-971.

Kannel, W. B.: Update on the role of cigarette smoking in coronary artery disease. Am Heart J 101, 1981, pp. 319-328.

Kramsch, D. M., Aspen, A. J., Abramowitz, B. M., Kreimendahl, T., and Hood, W. B. Jr.: Reduction of coronary atherosclerosis by moderate conditioning exercise in monkeys on an atherogenic diet. New Engl J Med 101, 1981, pp. 319-328.

Medical Letter: Oral contraceptives and the risk of cardiovascular disease. 25, 1983, pp. 69-70.

Neufeld, H. N. and Goldbourt, U.: Coronary heart disease: Genetic aspects. Circulation 67, 1983, pp. 943-954.

Review Panel in Coronary-Prone Behavior and Coronary Heart Disease: Coronary-prone behavior and coronary heart disease: A critical review. Circulation 63, 1981, pp. 1199-1215.

Roberts, W. C. and Waller, B. F.: Chronic hypercalcemia as a risk factor for coronary atherosclerosis. Cardiovasc Rev Rep 4, 1983, pp. 1275-1280.

Stadel, B. V.: Oral contraceptives and cardiovascular disease. N Engl J Med 305, 1981, pp. 612-618, 672-677.

PRIMARY AND SECONDARY PREVENTION
OF ATHEROSCLEROSIS

Ad Hoc Committee to Design a Dietary Treatment of Hyperlipoproteinemia, American Heart Association: AHA Special Report: Recommendations for treatment of hyperlipidemia in adults. Circulation 69, 1984, pp. 1065A-1090A.

Bethesda Conference Report. Eleventh Bethesda Conference: Prevention of coronary heart disease. Am J Cardiol 47, 1981, pp. 713-776.

Brensike, J. F., Levy, R. I., Kelsey, S. F., Passamani, E. R., Richardson, J. M., Loh, I. K., Stone, N. J., Aldrich, R. F., Battaglini, J. W., Moriarty, D. J., Fisher, M. R., Friedman, L., Friedwald, W., Detre, K. M., and Epstein, S. E.: Effects of therapy with cholestyramine in progression of coronary arteriosclerosis: results of the NHLBI Type II Coronary Intervention Study. Circulation 69, 1984, pp. 313-324.

Epstein, F. H. : Predicting, explaining, and preventing coronary heart disease. Mod Conc Cardiovasc Dis 48, 1979, pp. 7-12.

Fuchs, R. and Scheidt, S. S. : Prevention of coronary atherosclerosis. Cardiovasc Rev Rep 4, 1983, pp. 671-695, 691-812.

Gillum, R. F. , Folsom, A. , Luepker, R. V. , Jacobs, D. R. , Jr. , Kottke, T. E. , Gomez-Marin, O. , Prineas, R. J. , Taylor, H. L. , and Blackburn, H. : Sudden death and acute myocardial infarction in a metropolitan area, 1970-1980: The Minnesota Heart Survey. N Engl J Med 309, 1983, pp. 1353-1358.

Goldman, G. J. and Pichard, A. D. : The natural history of coronary artery disease: does medical therapy improve the prognosis? Prog Cardiovasc Dis 25, 1983, pp. 513-552.

Hammond, H. K. : Regression of atherosclerosis, a review. J Cardiol Rehab 3, 1983, pp. 347-359.

Hjermann, I. , Holme, I. , Byre, K. V., and Leren, P. : Effect of diet and smoking intervention on the incidence of coronary heart disease. Lancet 2, 1981, pp. 1303-1310.

Kannel, W. B. : Risk factors in established coronary heart disease: Prospects for secondary prevention, in McIntosh, H. D. (Ed.), "Baylor College of Medicine Cardiology Series," Vol. 4, 1981, pp. 7-25.

Kannel, W. B. : Prospects for risk factor modification to reduce risk of reinfarction and premature death. J Card Rehab 1, 1981, pp. 63-70.

Kornitzer, M. , DeBacker, G. , Dramaix, M. , and Thilly, C. : The Belgian Heart Disease Prevention Project. Modification of the coronary risk profile in an industrial population. Circulation 61, 1980, pp. 18-25.

Kuller, L. H. : Editorial: Prevention of cardiovascular disease and risk-factor intervention trials. Circulation 61, 1980, pp. 26-28.

Kuller, L. : Risk factor reduction in coronary heart disease. Mod Conc Cardiovasc Dis 53, 1984, pp. 7-11.

Kuo, P. T. , Wilson, A. C. , Goldstein, R. C. , and Schaub, R. G. : Suppression of experimental atherosclerosis in rabbits by interferon-inducing agents. J Am Coll Cardiol 3, 1984, pp. 129-134.

Levy, R. I. , Brensike, J. F. , Epstein, S. E. , Kelsey, S. F. , Passamani, E. R. , Richardson, J. M. , Loh, I. K. , Stone, N. J. , Aldrich, R. F. , Battaglini, J. W. , Moriarty, D. J. , Fisher, M. L. , Friedman, L. , Friedwald, W. , and Detre, K. M. : The influence of changes in lipid values induced by cholestyramine and diet on progression of coronary artery disease: results of the NHLBI Type II Coronary Intervention Study. Circulation 69, 1984, pp. 325-337.

Levy, R. I. : Progress toward prevention of cardiovascular disease. A thirty-year retrospective. Mod Conc Cardiovasc Dis 47, 1978, pp. 103-108.

Lewis, B. : Ischemic heart disease: The scientific basis, in Yu, P. N. and Goodwin, J. F. (Eds.), "Progress in Cardiology," Vol. 10, Lea & Febiger, Philadelphia, 1981, pp. 21-44.

Lipid Research Clinics Program: The Lipid Research Clinics Coronary Primary Prevention Trial Results: I. Reduction in incidence of coronary heart disease. JAMA 251, 1984, pp. 351-364.

Lipid Research Clinics Program: The Lipid Research Clinics Coronary Primary Prevention Trial Results. II. The relationship of reduction in incidence of coronary heart disease to cholesterol lowering. JAMA 251, 1984, pp. 365-374.

Malinow, M. R. : Regression of atherosclerosis in humans: Fact or myth? Circulation 64, 1981, pp. 1-3.

Meijler, F. I. : Prevention of coronary heart disease: A cardiologist's view, in Yu, P. N. and Goodwin, J. F. (Eds.), "Progress in Cardiology," Vol. 10, 1981, Lea & Febiger, Philadelphia, pp. 44-63.

Meijler, F. I. : Contribution of the risk factor concept to patient care in coronary heart disease. J Am Coll Cardiol 1, 1983, pp. 13-19.

Moser, M. : Clinical trials and their effect on medical therapy: The Multiple Risk Factor Intervention. Am Heart J 107, 1984, pp. 616-618.

Multiple Risk Factor Intervention Trial Research Group:
Multiple risk factor intervention trial. JAMA 248, 1982,
pp. 1465-1477.

Nash, D. T. and Gensini, G.: The progression of atherosclerosis. J Cardiac Rehab 4, 1984, pp. 21-26.

Oslo Study Research Group: MRFIT and the Oslo study. JAMA
249, 1983, pp. 893-894.

Singh, B. N. and Venkatesh, N.: Prevention of myocardial
reinfarction and of sudden death in survivors of acute myocardial infarction: role of prophylactic β-adrenoceptor blockade. Am Heart J 107, 1984, pp. 189-200.

Stamler, J.: Primary prevention of epidemic premature
atherosclerotic coronary heart disease, in Yu, P. N. and
Goodwin, J. F. (Eds.), "Progress in Cardiology," Vol. 10,
1981, Lea & Febiger, Philadelphia, pp. 63-100.

Stamler, J. and Stamler, R.: Intervention for the prevention
and control of hypertension and atherosclerotic diseases:
United States and international experience. Am J Med 76,
2/27/84, pp. 13-36.

Walker, W. J.: Changing U. S. life style and declining vascular
mortality - a retrospective. New Engl J Med 308, 1983, pp.
649-651.

Wilhelmsen, L.: Risk factors for coronary heart disease in
perspective. European Intervention trials. Am J Med 76,
2/27/84, pp. 37-40.

Zelis, R. F. and Wenger, N. K.: Prevention of coronary
atherosclerosis, in Hurst, J. W. (Ed.), "The Heart," 5th
Edition, McGraw-Hill, New York, 1982, pp. 959-976.

Chapter 12

CLINICAL CASE EXAMPLES

The following four case presentations are based on actual patient histories and are meant to be illustrative of typical clinical
presentations. Each section of the case presentation is followed
by a series of choices to be made, involving diagnostic and
therapeutic options. A discussion of these choices follows each
group of questions. The discussions are based upon information contained in various sections of the text.

CASE 1

PART A

A 27-year-old man comes to your office with a long history of
intermittently treated hypertension and now complains of recent
onset of substernal chest pressure which occurs when walking
a few blocks and also after eating a heavy meal. He has had no
pains at rest and no other symptoms. He smokes two packs of
cigarettes per day and states that his father died at age 60 of a
heart attack.

On examination he is slightly obese, has a blood pressure of
190/105 and a pulse of 85. The examination discloses the presence of a few xanthelasmas around the eyes and hypertensive
funduscopic changes. His cardiac examination reveals an S4
gallop sound.

His electrocardiogram shows normal sinus rhythm and QRS
and ST-T changes consistent with left ventricular hypertrophy.
A chest x-ray shows cardiomegaly without congestive changes.

Your first step in establishing a diagnosis and initiating
treatment would be (Choose one):

1. Perform a treadmill exercise test
2. Perform an upper GI series
3. Admit the patient to the hospital for a coronary angiogram
4. Start the patient on antihypertensive medication
5. Start the patient on nitroglycerin

Discussion

(1) Ordinarily, a treadmill exercise test would be among the first steps in evaluating a patient with exertional chest pain. In this case, however, there are two reasons why a treadmill exercise test should not be done at this point: first, severe hypertension is a contraindication to stress testing, since a submaximal or maximal stress test would increase blood pressure further to possibly dangerous levels. Second, one of the causes of a false-positive stress electrocardiogram is the presence of left ventricular hypertrophy on the electrocardiogram, and, therefore, a stress test in a patient with this electrocardiographic pattern would be impossible to interpret. (Although, the absence of electrocardiographic changes in response to exercise in the presence of left ventricular hypertrophy would still be valid as a negative stress test.)

(2) Ordering an upper GI series would also be inappropriate at this point in the workup, since the history is much more suggestive of the diagnosis of angina pectoris than of chest pain of gastrointestinal origin. The postprandial pattern of substernal pain can sometimes be indicative of a gastrointestinal origin of pain but is also frequently a sign of anginal pain, especially when it is also provoked by exertion. Moreover, the presence of multiple risk factors for atherosclerotic heart disease in this patient (hypertension, positive family history, smoking, and physical evidence of hypercholesterolemia, indicated by the presence of xanthelasmas) lends additional weight to the diagnosis of ischemic heart disease. Should further diagnostic workup not be consistent with the diagnosis of ischemic heart disease, an upper GI series might then be indicated.

(3) Coronary arteriography is the most definitive test for the diagnosis of coronary artery disease and in this case would be likely to confirm the clinical diagnosis of chest pain due to coronary artery disease. In addition, it would provide detailed information on the anatomy of the coronary lesions. Coronary arteriography would, therefore, be one appropriate approach to the diagnostic workup in this patient but would ordinarily be done either when other less invasive tests are inconclusive or suggest severe or critical coronary artery disease or when a definitive diagnosis must be made. In this case, performing a coronary arteriogram at this stage of the patient's workup and treatment would certainly be optional and would probably be left for a later time if clinically indicated.

(4) It would be most appropriate to start this patient on an antihypertensive medication in view of his severe hypertension as well as his apparent angina pectoris. Since hypertension is one

of the factors which increases myocardial oxygen consumption and thus increases angina, control of hypertension is mandatory in the acute treatment of angina pectoris as well as in the control of hypertension for prevention of chronic complications. Regardless of the ultimate form of treatment of this patient's chest pain, the first step in management is control of hypertension, which may be sufficient in itself to eliminate his symptoms of angina in the setting. The ideal choice of an antihypertensive drug would be a beta-blocker class of drug, which would not only control the hypertension but would also lower the heart rate and decrease myocardial contractility, all of which would decrease myocardial oxygen requirements and would be beneficial for the patient with ischemic heart disease and angina pectoris.

(5) The institution of nitroglycerin therapy for apparent angina pectoris is certainly appropriate. Sublingual nitroglycerin would be useful as a therapeutic test to confirm the diagnosis of angina as well as an important therapeutic modality. Immediate resolution of chest discomfort following nitroglycerin is important confirmatory evidence of the presence of angina pectoris. In addition, the use of nitroglycerin to relieve an episode of chest discomfort is the mainstay of therapy of angina pectoris. Prophylactic administration of nitroglycerin (prior to activity likely to provoke chest discomfort) is an equally important and appropriate use of this drug.

PART B

The patient has been started on a beta-blocker drug and has been given a trial of sublingual nitroglycerin to use to relieve an episode of chest discomfort and to take prior to exercise. He returns to your office a few days later reporting that the nitroglycerin did indeed relieve his chest discomfort promptly and when used in conjunction with the beta-blocker, has significantly reduced the frequency of his episodes of chest discomfort. However, he still has some discomfort with brisk walking or walking up an incline. His blood pressure is now found to be 160/95 and his resting pulse rate is 72 beats/min. At this point a diuretic is added to his treatment, and he returns a week later with a blood pressure of 140/85.

At this point you would:

1. Continue the current therapy and advise the patient to lose some weight and stop smoking
2. Add a long-acting nitrate preparation
3. Perform a stress electrocardiogram
4. Perform a thallium stress test

Discussion

(1) Certainly answer (1) is appropriate, since medical therapy has thus far been successful and weight loss and discontinuation of smoking are valuable in control of hypertension as well as in preventing the complications of coronary artery disease.

(2) Addition of a long-acting nitrate drug would also be appropriate at this point to further reduce the incidence of angina pectoris. Any of the currently available forms of long-acting nitroglycerin would be appropriate, and ordinarily, a low dose should be started to determine the patient's tolerance to this type of drug, and the dose can subsequently be increased as necessary to achieve adequate control of symptoms. A long-acting nitrate drug would also help to control his hypertension.

(3) For the reason discussed in Part A, a routine stress electrocardiographic test may be difficult to interpret because of the presence of left ventricular hypertrophy but would serve a useful purpose in determining the patient's exercise tolerance and, more specifically, the heart rate and blood pressure response to exercise and the heart rate-blood pressure product at which angina develops. This would allow better determination of the efficacy of drug therapy and would also provide some indication as to the severity of the coronary artery disease.

(4) A thallium stress test would be even more useful than a routine electrocardiographic stress test, since it would also provide additional information on myocardial perfusion abnormalities with exercise and would provide the confirmatory evidence of the presence of ischemic heart disease as well as information on the extent and distribution of the coronary disease. A thallium stress test may provide an alternative to coronary arteriography at this point in the patient's management, since it should distinguish mild or limited coronary artery disease from severe or extensive coronary artery disease. Although a thallium stress test is generally most helpful in cases where the diagnosis of coronary artery disease is in doubt, this test is also highly useful in providing prognostic information for an individual patient and aids in determining which patients should be considered for coronary arteriography and possible coronary bypass surgery.

PART C

A decision is made to perform a thallium stress test prior to increasing his medication. The test is performed while the patient is taking his current dose of beta-blocker medication, and he is able to complete three stages of a standard Bruce

protocol stress test (9 minutes of exercise) and develops substernal pressure during the last minute of exercise at which
time his heart rate is 140 and his blood pressure is 175/90.
Within one minute of discontinuing exercise, his chest discomfort has disappeared and his heart rate has decreased to
85. The electrocardiogram shows the development of 2 mm of
additional ST segment depression (compared to the resting
ECG) at peak exercise, which gradually returns to baseline and
is most marked in the inferior leads. The thallium images
show decreased perfusion along the inferior wall of the left
ventricle at peak exercise with normalization in the redistribution images taken 4 hours later. There is no evidence of abnormal increased pulmonary uptake of thallium during exercise.
    At this point you recommend:

1. A nuclear wall motion study
2. Coronary arteriography
3. Continuation of the current medical therapy
4. An increase in the dosage of the beta-blocker
5. Obtaining a serum cholesterol level and initiating treat-
    ment if hypercholesterolemia is found

Discussion

(1) An exercise wall motion study would not be likely to add further additional useful information for the diagnosis and management of the patient at this point, since the diagnosis of coronary
artery disease has essentially been confirmed by the thallium
stress test. It is likely that a wall motion study would show abnormalities in wall motion during exercise corresponding to the
areas of abnormality shown by the thallium stress test. Furthermore, it would add additional expense to the workup.
    (2) Coronary arteriography would be expected to confirm the
diagnosis of obstructive coronary artery disease in this patient
and would further define the exact anatomy of the disease. A
major indication for performing coronary arteriography in this
setting would be to evaluate the patient for the possibility of
left main coronary artery disease or severe multivessel disease,
either of which might be a basis for recommending coronary
artery bypass surgery in symptomatic patients. Another reason
for performing coronary arteriography in a patient with angina
pectoris would be to evaluate the patient for the possibility of
coronary angioplasty, providing the patient was severely symptomatic. In this case, the thallium stress test suggests that his
disease is limited to the coronary supply to the inferior wall of
the left ventricle, which is usually a result of right coronary

artery disease. If the patient had left main coronary artery disease or severe multivessel disease, he would be expected to show more widespread thallium perfusion abnormalities. Since the patient has not yet received maximum medical therapy, consideration for bypass surgery or coronary angioplasty based on symptomatology is not warranted at this point.

(3) The patient has had a good clinical response to the current medical therapy, but he is still somewhat limited by angina, and his stress thallium test documented ischemia at a relatively low pulse rate, suggesting that his medical therapy is probably not yet optimal.

(4) On the current medical regimen his resting pulse rate is in the 70s, his resting blood pressure is 140/85, and his exercise heart rate is found to be 140 with an exercise blood pressure of 175/90. In view of both the resting and exercise heart rate and blood pressure, there is still room to increase his beta-blocker dose. The usual guideline for adjusting beta-blocker dosages is to achieve a resting pulse rate of 55 to 65 and a maximum heart rate with exercise of approximately 130 (or below the pressure at which angina occurs), without decreasing the blood pressure to the point where the patient develops orthostatic hypotension or decreased coronary artery perfusion.

(5) It is highly likely that this patient has hypercholesterolemia, based on the fact that he has evidence of coronary artery disease at a relatively young age as well as a positive family history of coronary disease and the presence of xanthelasmas on examination. With the recent evidence that secondary prevention of ischemic heart disease is practical by utilization of cholesterol modification in patients with hypercholesterolemia, means to achieve reduction in serum cholesterol in this patient are certainly indicated if he indeed does have hypercholesterolemia.

PART D

The patient's dose of beta-blocker medication is increased, and he is started on a long-acting nitrate preparation such that his resting heart rate is now approximately 60 and resting blood pressure 125/70. He now finds that he is able to resume all of his activities without angina, although he still avoids particularly strenuous activities out of concern for his condition. He is found to have a serum cholesterol of 320 mg%, and he is instructed on a low-cholesterol diet and a repeat serum cholesterol done 2 months later is down to 260 mg%.

He continues to do well clinically, with only occasional angina pains, until about a year later, at which time he starts to have a recurrence of his angina, which becomes increasingly more frequent despite continued good control of his blood pressure and heart rate with combination of a beta-blocker drug and a nitrate drug. A decision is made at this point to perform coronary arteriography. The left ventriculogram shows a normal left ventricular contraction pattern. The left coronary artery shows approximately 40% narrowing in the mid-left anterior descending artery and some irregularities in the circumflex coronary arteries but no significant obstructive lesion in this vessel. The right coronary artery has a 95% proximal occlusive lesion. Despite continued adherence to his low-cholesterol diet, a serum cholesterol is repeated and found to be 285 mg%. At this point you recommend:

1. Coronary artery bypass surgery
2. Percutaneous transluminal coronary angioplasty
3. Addition of a calcium channel blocking agent
4. Addition of a cholesterol-lowering agent
5. Curtailment of his activity level to reduce the amount of angina pectoris

Discussion

(1) Coronary artery disease bypass surgery would not be recommended in this case due to essentially single-vessel coronary artery disease which should be amenable to angioplasty (PTCA). In a patient of this age, particularly with evidence of disease developing in the left anterior descending coronary artery, surgery should be postponed until absolutely necessary.

(2) This would appear to be an excellent situation for percutaneous transluminal coronary angioplasty. Dilatation of the proximal right coronary artery lesion, if successful, should essentially alleviate the patient's angina and ischemia and postpone the need for surgery.

(3) An alternative to PTCA would be the addition of a calcium channel blocking agent to the patient's regimen. Certainly this could be tried prior to the time of PTCA, and in certain cases significant reduction in effort angina will be achieved. If significant alleviation of angina does not occur with the addition of a calcium channel blocking agent, then PTCA certainly should be done at this point.

(4) Regardless of any other therapeutic modality being undertaken, it would be appropriate to add a cholesterol-lowering agent such as one of the bile sequestrating drugs. Certainly this would be more of a long-term than short-term therapeutic modality and would have no immediate impact on the patient's symptoms.

(5) Curtailment of physical activity is certainly one method of reducing angina pectoris but would not be likely to be an acceptable alternative to this fairly young man when other effective measures are available.

DISCUSSION OF CASE 1

This case represents a fairly typical example of a patient with multiple risk factors for coronary artery disease, whose angina pectoris is very easily controllable with control of his blood pressure and the use of antianginal medication. His thallium test suggested single-vessel disease in the right coronary artery distribution, and this was subsequently confirmed by coronary arteriography. He eventually failed to respond to medical therapy and was found to have a high-grade proximal right coronary artery lesion which was suitable for percutaneous transluminal coronary angioplasty. He was also found to have hypercholesterolemia, only partially responsive to diet, and required treatment with a cholesterol-lowering agent. It would be anticipated that such a patient would benefit from angioplasty and cholesterol reduction but would probably have progressive arteriosclerosis which may require subsequent angioplasties in the same or other arteries or perhaps coronary artery bypass surgery at some point.

CASE 2

PART A

A 64-year-old man with stable exertional angina pectoris previously well controlled on a beta-blocker medication and a long-acting nitrate medication informs you that over the past few weeks he has been getting his anginal pains much more frequently and with less effort and has even been having some pain at rest on occasion. His nitroglycerin use has increased considerably. There are no obvious predisposing factors to his increased angina such as increased emotional or physical stress. Upon examination, his heart rate is 62, his blood pressure is 124/68, and he has no significant abnormal findings. His resting electrocardiogram is unchanged from his usual electrocardiogram, which is essentially normal.

Your response at this point would be to:

1. Hospitalize the patient for observation and further management
2. Recommend coronary arteriography

3. Increase the beta-blocker and/or nitrate medications
4. Add a calcium channel blocking agent
5. Perform a submaximal treadmill stress test

Discussion

(1) This patient has had a recent change in his previously stable angina pectoris and therefore fits into the category of unstable angina pectoris. The usual approach to such a patient would be to admit him to the hospital for observation and further management. While in the hospital, his heart rate and electrocardiogram could be continuously monitored and his blood pressure could be checked frequently. Modified bed rest would be recommended for the first few days to "cool off" the patient, with subsequent gradual ambulation. If an episode of angina occurred in this setting, the blood pressure and heart rate response as well as the electrocardiographic pattern could be evaluated to provide the physician with guidelines for the choice of additional medication. An episode of angina associated with an increase in blood pressure and heart rate and accompanying ST segment depression on the electrocardiogram would suggest that the anginal episodes are occurring as a result of increased oxygen demand and would likely be responsive to increased doses of beta-blocker and/or nitrate medication. Since the patient is in the hospital, the doses could be increased as frequently as necessary, since vital signs and symptoms are being carefully observed. If anginal episodes occur without a significant change in blood pressure or heart rate, and the electrocardiogram shows ST depression or elevation, it is likely that the episodes are related to occurrences of increased coronary artery tone (spasm) and thus result from decreased coronary flow rather than from increased oxygen demand. In such a case, the treatment of choice would be either a nitrate drug (in high dose) or a calcium channel blocking agent to prevent this increased tone. The beta-blocker might also be carefully decreased while the calcium channel blocking drug is being added if coronary artery spasm is suspected, since beta-blockers may increase coronary tone. Having the patient remain in the hospital would then allow assessment of the response to therapy as the patient's activity level is increased.

(2) Coronary arteriography would be indicated in this patient, since he very likely has "critical" coronary artery disease and possibly has left main coronary artery disease. Knowledge of the patient's coronary anatomy would be helpful in further decisions regarding therapy as well as in providing prognostic information. In this particular case, coronary arteriography

could be done early in the patient's management with subsequent
optimization of medical therapy if the patient is not felt to be a
surgical candidate, or it could be done subsequent to in-hospital
medical management, as discussed above.

(3) Either or both of these agents could be increased, but
since the patient's resting heart rate and blood pressure are already in an optimal range, it is questionable whether further increases in either of these medications would be either well tolerated or markedly effective. In a hospital setting, however,
either or both of these agents could be further increased to the
point of tolerance or effectiveness in an attempt to get the patient
through his current episode of unstable angina.

(4) Addition of a calcium channel blocking agent at this point
would certainly be an alternative to any of the above approaches.
Many patients with unstable angina pectoris do respond to the
addition of a calcium channel blocking agent, regardless of
whether or not the increase in angina is secondary to increased
coronary tone. Again, the addition of this drug would best be
done in a hospital setting because of this patient's unstable
status, but if for some reason it was not feasible to hospitalize
the patient at this point, the addition of this agent could be done
on an outpatient basis if the patient could be monitored closely.
If the calcium channel blocking drug resulted in excessive reduction in the heart rate or blood pressure, as can occur, this
could conceivably result in a worsening rather than an improvement in the patient's angina. Selection of the appropriate
calcium channel blocking drug as well as close observation of
the patient during his initial period of treatment with this type
of drug should help to avoid this potential complication.

(5) Unstable angina pectoris is a definite contraindication to
treadmill exercise testing. An exercise test in this setting is
likely to provoke a severe episode of angina pectoris or coronary insufficiency or even acute myocardial infarction, without providing any necessary information for the patient's
management.

PART B

The patient is admitted to the hospital for observation as suggested. His initial electrocardiogram is shown in Figure
12-1A. While at rest, the patient has a spontaneous episode of
chest pain and a repeat electrocardiogram is taken (Figure
12-1B). Between the time of the first and second electrocardiogram, his heart rate has increased from 62 to 72 beats/
min, and his blood pressure has increased from 118/70 to
154/80. He was immediately given a sublingual tablet of

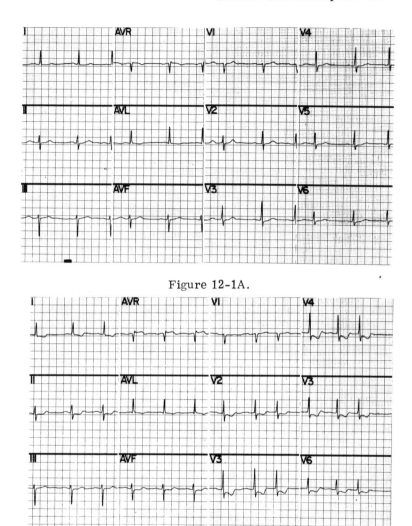

Figure 12-1A.

Figure 12-1B.

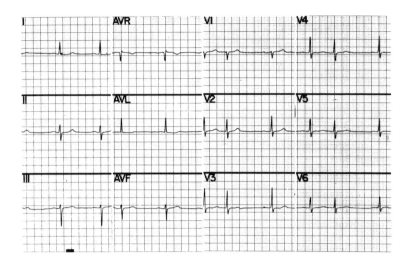

Figure 12-1C.

nitroglycerin and his pain resolved within a few minutes. A
repeat electrocardiogram was done at this point and is illustrated in Figure 12-1C.
  You now advise:

  1. Further increase in the patient's current medications
      to the point of tolerance
  2. Immediate coronary arteriography
  3. Addition of a calcium channel blocking agent
  4. Initiation of an intravenous drip of nitroglycerin
  5. Insertion of an intraaortic balloon counterpulsation
      device

Discussion

(1) Despite bed rest and good levels of resting blood pressure and
pulse rate, this patient experiences spontaneous episodes of
angina pectoris accompanied by increases in blood pressure and
heart rate and marked ST segment abnormalities on the electrocardiogram. The widespread distribution of ST segment changes
on the electrocardiogram would indicate extensive or even
global ischemia. Additional increase in the dose of the beta-
blocker drug as well as the nitrate drug that the patient has
been on may help to prevent further such episodes but are
probably insufficient measures in this case.

(2) Coronary arteriography would definitely be indicated in this patient, since it is likely that he has severe coronary artery disease and may require coronary artery bypass surgery.

(3) A calcium channel blocking agent would also be of a potential benefit in this type of patient and should be tried at this time. However, it is unlikely that this will be sufficiently effective to significantly alter the course of this patient, who most likely has severe arteriosclerotic disease.

(4) An intravenous drip of nitroglycerin would definitely be indicated in this patient, since this is the most effective form of nitroglycerin in patients with unstable angina pectoris and allows precise control on a moment-to-moment basis, while following the patient's arterial blood pressure and clinical state. The availability of this modality of treatment is one of the reasons for hospitalizing such patients.

(5) Intraaortic balloon counterpulsation is certainly an effective method for preventing episodes of rest angina but would not be indicated at this point in the patient's management. Should the patient continue having episodes of rest angina while on an effective dose of intravenous nitroglycerin as well as effective doses of beta-blocker and calcium blocking drugs, then this modality would be indicated until such time as the patient can undergo coronary arteriography and definitive treatment.

PART C

The patient is started on a nitroglycerin infusion and has no further episodes of chest pain or electrocardiographic changes. On the following day the patient undergoes coronary arteriography and is found to have severe three-vessel coronary artery disease, with subtotal occlusions of the proximal segments of each of the major coronary arteries, with a good caliber of the vessels beyond the sites of proximal obstruction. The left ventriculogram shows normal contraction. At this point you would advise:

1. Gradually tapering the nitroglycerin infusion and switch the patient over to effective doses of oral and/or topical preparations
2. Immediate coronary artery bypass surgery
3. Percutaneous transluminal coronary angioplasty (PTCA)
4. The patient to alter his life-style to avoid activities that may precipitate the anginal episodes

Discussion

(1) Although the patient may be able to get through his current episode of unstable angina pectoris and return to his previous

pattern, it is unlikely that a patient with this degree of coronary artery disease would continue to do well on a long-term basis and would most likely have recurrent episodes of unstable angina pectoris or acute myocardial infarction. This approach, therefore, would not be recommended.

(2) Given this patient's symptomatology and his angiographic findings, coronary artery bypass surgery is the treatment of choice and should be done as soon as feasible. The patient should be maintained on the intravenous nitroglycerin until the time of surgery. If he has further episodes of angina pectoris despite an adequate dose of intravenous nitroglycerin, an intra-aortic balloon counterpulsation device might need to be inserted prior to surgery to provide extra protection to the patient during the perioperative period.

(3) With severe three-vessel coronary artery disease, PTCA would not be recommended at this time, since surgery is more likely to result in a long-term successful outcome.

(4) This approach would certainly be inadequate in a patient this age and with this degree of coronary artery disease. This approach would only be recommended for patients with inoperable disease or patients who refuse surgery and are having angina primarily with physical activity.

PART D

The patient undergoes coronary artery bypass surgery to all affected vessels as you have recommended. He has a benign course and is subsequently relieved of all anginal pains and is able to return to a normal life-style off all cardiac medication. A treadmill exercise test done 6 months after surgery shows excellent exercise tolerance without development of angina pectoris or ST segment abnormalities.

DISCUSSION OF CASE 2

This case represents a fairly typical example of unstable angina pectoris due to severe multivessel coronary artery disease in which symptoms can be controlled temporarily with the use of intravenous nitroglycerin. Due to the severe nature of the disease, however, surgical therapy is most likely to provide the patient with long-term and effective relief of his symptoms and may, in selective situations, decrease the likelihood of subsequent myocardial infarction and complications.

CASE 3

PART A

A 58-year-old woman without a prior history of cardiac problems is brought to the hospital emergency room with a 4-5-hour history of severe, crushing-type chest pain, shortness of breath, and nausea. Upon examination, she is pale, mildly cyanotic, diaphoretic, and tachypneic, with a respiratory rate of 36/minute, a blood pressure of 90/55, and a pulse rate of 90. Her neck veins are distended, even in the sitting position, and on examination of the chest, rales are heard two-thirds of the way up bilaterally. Her heart sounds are soft, there is a grade 4/6 holosystolic blowing murmur best heart at the apex and there is an S3 gallop. Her extremities are cool, and there is no peripheral edema.

The electrocardiogram is illustrated in Figure 12-2. The chest x-ray shows an enlarged heart and pulmonary congestion. Your first steps would include:

1. Administration of oxygen and morphine
2. Rapid administration of fluid intravenously
3. Administration of a diuretic intravenously
4. Placement of a flow-directed pulmonary artery (Swan-Ganz) catheter
5. Administration of streptokinase (given by either intracoronary or intravenous injection)

Discussion

(1) Administration of oxygen is certainly indicated, especially in the presence of tachypnea, cyanosis, and continuing chest pain. A high flow face mask would be indicated for pulmonary congestion and cyanosis. Morphine sulphate would also be indicated for severe chest pain and pulmonary edema and would have to be given in small doses in view of the borderline hypotension to avoid further hypotension.

(2) Rapid administration of intravenous fluids would certainly be contraindicated in the presence of obvious congestive heart failure, despite the low blood pressure. A trial of intravenous fluid would be appropriate to raise a low blood pressure in the absence of signs of heart failure, however.

(3) Administration of an intravenous diuretic would certainly be called for in the presence of severe congestive heart failure. However, the blood pressure would have to be monitored closely, since it could potentially fall as a result of rapid diuresis if the

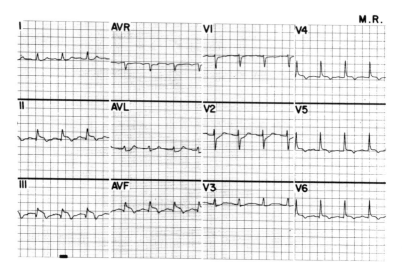

Figure 12-2.

heart requires a high left ventricular filling pressure to maintain a cardiac output sufficient to keep the blood pressure in a normal range.

(4) The insertion of a flow-directed pulmonary artery catheter is indicated in critically ill patients with acute myocardial infarction, especially when hypotension occurs in conjunction with congestive heart failure, to allow more rational choice of treatment as well as to follow the patient's condition and response to therapy more closely. This procedure should be done as soon as feasible but should not interfere with other urgent therapeutic steps.

(5) The electrocardiogram clearly shows an acute inferior-lateral myocardial infarction with Q wave and ST segment elevations in leads 2, 3, AVF, and V_2-V_6. Administration of streptokinase is rapidly becoming a standard part of the treatment of acute myocardial infarction to reopen a thrombosed coronary artery and to reestablish blood supply to an ischemic myocardium to limit the ultimate size of the myocardial infarction. In this case, the time from onset of symptoms (4-5 hours) is slightly beyond the optimal time of 3 hours or less for maximal effectiveness of this treatment, and the presence of Q waves would indicate that myocardial necrosis has already occurred. It still may be worth trying this approach, however, if the initiation of this treatment does not delay other necessary treatment. At the present time, the most extensive experience

is with intracoronary injection of streptokinase, and this is the only method of administration which is currently approved for use by the FDA. Intravenous streptokinase is currently undergoing therapeutic trials to compare the efficacy to the intracoronary method, and certainly the intravenous approach is much simpler and faster and much more practical. If this is shown to be as effective as intracoronary streptokinase, then it is likely that this will become a standard form of therapy of acute myocardial infarction in the early stages.

PART B

Steps 1, 3, and 4 are initiated. It was elected not to give streptokinase because it was felt that it would delay other more essential therapy and also because of the concern of the possible bleeding complications during the insertion of the pulmonary artery catheter. A Foley catheter was also inserted to monitor urine output, and arterial blood gases were obtained. Initial data were as follows:

Arterial blood gases (on O_2 mask): pH 7.29, PO_2 66 mmHg, PCO_2 41 mmHg, HCO_3 19 mEq/L, O_2 saturation 91%.

Urine output: initially 20 cc in the first hour, then (following intravenous furosemide) 150 cc the next hour.

Hemodynamics:

     Right atrium: mean = 12 mmHg (normal = 2-8)
     Pulmonary artery 45/24 (normal = 15-30/4-12)
     Pulmonary capillary wedge: mean = 20 mmHg (normal = 6-12), "a" wave = 18 mmHg, "v" wave = 35 mmHg (normal "a" = 3-15, normal "v" = 3-15)
     Cardiac output = 3.2 M/min, cardiac index = 1.9 L/min/M^2 (normal cardiac output = 3.5-7, normal cardiac index = 2.5-4.0)
     Arterial pressure = 98/60, systemic vascular resistance = 1900 dynes-sec-cm^{-5} (normal = 900-1400)

There was no step up in oxygen saturation between the right ventricle and right atrium.

At this point, the patient's cyanosis is improved, but she is still in moderate respiratory distress and still has cool and clammy extremities. Your next step would be to administer:

1.   More intravenous furosemide
2.   More intravenous fluid
3.   A vasodilator

4. A vasopressor
5. A positive inotropic agent

Discussion

(1) Additional diuresis would be helpful to reduce the pulmonary capillary wedge pressure, and thus to improve the patient's respiratory status, but would be somewhat risky as sole therapy in view of a low cardiac output, since a high left ventricular filling pressure would be necessary to maintain cardiac output in a failing heart. Reducing the filling pressure without improving cardiac function at the same time may therefore be detrimental.

(2) Giving additional intravenous fluid would certainly not be indicated in view of the high pulmonary capillary wedge pressure. Having this information from a pulmonary artery flow directed catheter provides this very useful guideline, which might be difficult to deduce correctly from clinical means only.

(3) Despite the mild systemic hypotension, a vasodilator would be indicated for the treatment of congestive heart failure, as well as for improvement of cardiac output in the presence of increased systemic vascular resistance and for the reduction of mitral regurgitation, which is diagnosed by the presence of the holosystolic murmur and the large "v" waves in the pulmonary capillary wedge pressure tracing. A holosystolic murmur might also be indicative of a ruptured ventricular septum, but the lack of oxygen saturation step-up in the right ventricle, as well as the large "v" waves in the pulmonary capillary wedge tracing, establishes that the murmur is due to mitral regurgitation rather than to a septal rupture. A rapidly acting intravenous vasodilator that can be titrated carefully should be used, such as nitroprusside. The dose is determined by the clinical and hemodynamic responses. With an improved cardiac output and decreased mitral regurgitation, systolic arterial pressures should increase rather than decrease.

(4) A vasoconstrictor is contraindicated despite the low blood pressure because of high systemic vascular resistance and the presence of mitral regurgitation. Further dose of vasoconstriction would tend to increase the amount of mitral regurgitation and to decrease the cardiac output further. Vasoconstrictors should be used only when the hypotension is associated with a normal or reduced systemic vascular resistance.

(5) A positive inotropic agent (dopamine or dobutamine) would not be the first choice of therapy, even though reduced left ventricular contraction may be partially responsible for the

problems of congestive heart failure and hypotension. As
indicated in the above discussion, a vasodilator would be the
first choice. However, if cardiac output failed to improve
adequately with vasodilator therapy, one of these positive
inotropic drugs might be used in conjunction with a vasodilator
to improve cardiac output if clinically indicated.

PART C

A nitroprusside intravenous infusion is initiated, with subsequent
clinical improvement in that the patient is no longer dyspneic
and her color is improved and urine output is increased. Her
chest pain is also improved, and the electrocardiogram shows
some resolution of the ST segment abnormalities. Repeat
arterial blood gases (on oxygen) now show the following:
ph = 7.41, pO_2 = 96 mmHg, pCO_2 = 34 mmHg, HCO_3 = 25 mEq/L.

Hemodynamics now show:

> Right atrium = 10 mmHg
> Pulmonary artery = 36/18 mmHg
> Pulmonary capillary wedge pressure = mean 18 mmHg,
>   a waves = 14 and v waves = 20 mmHg
> Arterial blood pressure = 100/70 mmHg
> Cardiac output = 4.8 liters/min
> Cardiac index = 3.0 liters/min/M^2
> SVR = 1,458 dynes sec/cm^{-5}

The electrocardiogram is repeated and is shown in Figure 12-3.
You would now:

1. Give lidocaine intravenously
2. Give atropine intravenously
3. Insert a temporary transvenous pacemaker
4. Check the blood pressure and clinical state of the patient
   and inform the nurse to observe the monitor closely for
   further changes

Discussion

(1) The electrocardiogram now shows the development of second
degree atrioventricular block of the type I (Wenckebach) variety,
which is a common complication of inferior wall myocardial infarction. The irregular R-R intervals are a consequence of this
conduction abnormality and not of premature beats. Lidocaine
would be strongly contraindicated, as the patient may develop

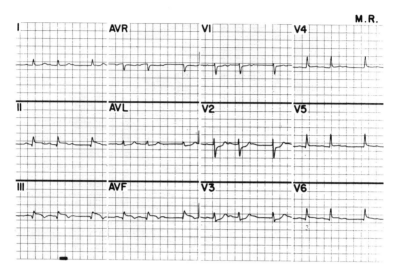

Figure 12-3.

complete heart block, and lidocaine would tend to suppress escape rhythms.

(2) Atropine is usually effective in reversing the heart block associated with inferior wall myocardial infarction but would not usually be given at this point, since the rhythm is not likely to cause any hemodynamic compromise. Furthermore, in this case the atrial rate is 100, and atropine is likely to further increase this rate, which could have two possible adverse effects:

a. Development of sinus tachycardia, which would increase myocardial oxygen consumption and might produce further ischemia and infarct extension.

b. If the atropine effect is greater on the sinoatrial node than on the atrioventricular node, the increase in sinus rate may convert a Wenckebach rhythm to a higher degree A-V block so that the ventricular rate may slow excessively.

(3) Insertion of a temporary transvenous pacemaker into the right ventricle would avoid the problems associated with atropine and would provide more controlled and longer duration of protection against bradycardia than would atropine. However, a pacemaker is optional at this point if the patient's status is otherwise stable, since second degree A-V block is often

transient in inferior wall myocardial infarction. Furthermore, ventricular pacing is likely to cause further hemodynamic compromise, since there would be loss of the atrial kick of sinus rhythm.

(4) Careful observation is the treatment of choice if the patient's hemodynamic and clinical conditions are stable in second degree heart block and the setting is such that a temporary pacemaker can be inserted quickly at any time if the block becomes more advanced or if the patient's condition deteriorates. The development of second degree A-V block (usually not of the type I or Wenckebach variety) in association with an anterior (rather than inferior) wall myocardial infarction is of different significance and is managed differently, since in this setting, development of third degree AV block is likely and is usually associated with slow ventricular escape rates and usually with extensive myocardial infarction.

PART D

The second degree A-V block spontaneously resolves without the need for a pacemaker or atropine. An attempt is made to discontinue the nitroprusside infusion, but whenever the infusion is reduced in order to discontinue it, the patient becomes more dyspneic and develops more chest pain and recurrent ST segment depression in the anterior leads, and the mitral regurgitation murmur becomes louder and the hemodynamics deteriorate.

At this point you would:

1.   Continue the nitroprusside as long as necessary
2.   Attempt to switch the patient to an oral or topical vasodilator drug
3.   Recommend cardiac catheterization and coronary arteriography for the consideration of possible surgery
4.   Perform a radionuclide wall motion study (resting, bedside) or a two-dimensional echocardiogram
5.   Insert an intraaortic balloon counterpulsation pump

Discussion

(1) Once successful therapy is begun, it is often difficult to know when to discontinue such treatment, but in the case of any intravenous therapy, it is a temporizing measure, meant to be used until more definitive treatment can be instituted. In this case, definitive therapy may be an oral or topical vasodilator, or possible surgery, or perhaps just time, to allow the acute event to stabilize.

(2) Normally this would be the approach to take. The nitro-prusside would be gradually tapered and subsequently discontinued, while at the same time an oral vasodilator such as hydralazine or prazosin is started. A venodilator, in the form of an oral or topical nitrate, would probably be of benefit as well to reduce preload in conjunction with a diuretic. The pulmonary artery (and peripheral artery) catheters would be left in place during this process, if possible, to allow accurate monitoring of the hemodynamic efficacy of the substitute therapy.

(3) There are two possible indications for surgery in this patient—one is the evidence of significant myocardial ischemia in addition to the acute myocardial infarction, based upon the recurrence of chest pain and ST segment depression in the anterior leads. Continued ischemia (especially if in a different electrocardiographic area from the acute infarction) is associated with a poor immediate and long-term prognosis. In this case, the ST segment depression seen in leads V_1-V_3 may indicate anterior wall ischemia ("ischemia at a distance") or may represent true posterior wall acute injury in association with inferior wall infarction. When it is necessary to use continuous intravenous nitroprusside to control the ischemia and heart failure, coronary artery bypass surgery may be necessary in the acute phase of myocardial infarction rather than as an elective procedure after recovery. The second reason for considering early surgery is the presence of hemodynamically significant mitral regurgitation resulting in heart failure. In this case, the degree of mitral regurgitation is variable, relating to the degree of systemic vascular resistance and also to the degree of ischemia, suggesting that the etiology is papillary muscle dysfunction rather than a ruptured papillary muscle or ruptured chordae tendinae. Therefore, early cardiac catheterization and coronary angiography is indicated both to quantitate the degree of mitral regurgitation (by left ventricular contrast angiography) and to delineate the coronary anatomy to determine the appropriateness of coronary bypass surgery.

(4) A noninvasive test for the assessment of left ventricular function such as a nuclear wall motion study or a two-dimensional echocardiogram would help to determine whether the patient's congestive heart failure and low cardiac output are primarily on the basis of left ventricular dysfunction, mitral regurgitation, or a combination of both, since further decisions on therapy would be based on this differentiation. Left ventricular and right ventricular ejection fractions and regional wall motion can be readily assessed, and an estimation of the degree of mitral regurgitation can also be assessed using the nuclear wall motion study. Two-dimensional echocardiography would

provide the same information as well as a measurement of chamber sizes. In addition, it would allow rapid assessment of the effect of changing interventions, since repeat and serial bedside studies are easily accomplished.

(5) The insertion of an intraaortic balloon counterpulsation device may be indicated to stabilize the patient if the myocardial ischemia and/or the mitral regurgitation cannot be controlled adequately with medical therapy, particularly if surgical treatment is being considered. Intraaortic balloon counterpulsation accomplishes two goals—it reduces arterial afterload and also increases coronary perfusion, both of which would be beneficial in the patient with ongoing ischemia, left ventricular dysfunction, and mitral regurgitation. It is particularly useful in stabilizing patients prior to and following cardiac surgery. In this patient, the use of this modality would be reserved for failure of medical therapy or for preparation for surgery.

PART E

A nuclear wall motion study is performed while the patient is on a nitroprusside infusion and shows a right ventricular ejection fraction of 40%, and a left ventricular ejection fraction of 35%, with akinesis of the inferior and posterior lateral walls and hypokinesis of the anterolateral wall and apex. The interventricular septum contracts normally. A two-dimensional echocardiogram is also performed and shows mild left atrial enlargement and left ventricular enlargement. A repeat study performed during a spontaneous episode of chest pain shows further left ventricular and left atrial enlargement and worsening of the wall motion abnormalities in the anterolateral wall and apex. Despite continued and increasing doses of nitroprusside, the patient still has episodes of angina with corresponding transient worsening of left ventricular function. A decision is made to insert an intraaortic balloon counterpulsation device and to proceed with coronary arteriography and left ventricular catheterization. The patient is stabilized and these procedures are performed.

The left ventriculogram demonstrates moderately severe mitral regurgitation in addition to the previously noted wall motion abnormalities. The coronary arteriogram shows total obstruction of the proximal circumflex coronary artery and subtotal occlusion of the mid-right coronary artery and a high-grade lesion of the proximal left anterior descending coronary artery. There are collateral blood vessels from the left anterior descending vessel to the circumflex artery. A decision is made to perform surgery, and the patient undergoes successful triple bypass surgery and mitral valve replacement.

Following this she does well, without further chest pain or congestive heart failure.

DISCUSSION OF CASE 3

This case illustrates several of the many potential complications of acute myocardial infarction as well as the use of some of the techniques used to diagnose these complications and examples of modes of therapy which are available. Although many cases of heart failure and hypotension associated with acute myocardial infarction are due to cardiogenic shock as a result of extensive myocardial necrosis and are not responsive to medical or surgical therapy, cases with reversible causes need to be quickly identified and appropriately treated.

CASE 4

PART A

A 41-year-old female comes to you complaining of recent onset of chest pains. The pain is located in the substernal and left anterior chest areas and is described as a pressure-like sensation. It is not necessarily associated with activity or eating and usually lasts for a few minutes at a time. She also notes episodes of palpitations and light-headedness which often accompany the chest pain. There is no family history of early coronary artery disease or known hypercholesterolemia.

On examination, her blood pressure is 125/70, her pulse rate is 68 and regular, and her examination is entirely unremarkable except for a grade 1-2/6 soft systolic murmur at the apex and lower left sternal border.

The resting electrocardiogram, chest x-ray, and routine laboratory data including serum cholesterol are all within normal limits. A treadmill stress test is done, and the patient exercises for 12 minutes on the Bruce protocol without chest pain and reaches a heart rate of 176 beats/min. The electrocardiogram shows 1 mm of upsloping ST segment depression at peak exercise.

At this point, you would:

1. Give the patient an empiric trial of nitroglycerin to be used for episodes of chest pain
2. Start the patient on a beta-blocker drug
3. Order a thallium stress test
4. Perform coronary fluoroscopy
5. Order an echocardiogram

Discussion

(1) Whenever a diagnosis of angina pectoris is considered, an empiric trial of nitroglycerin is usually worthwhile. A dramatic response of the chest pain to nitroglycerin with relief within 1 to 2 minutes is convincing evidence for a coronary basis for the chest pains (with the exception of an esophageal spasm, which may also respond to nitroglycerin). Moreover, with the possible exception of hypotension (especially orthostatic), nitroglycerin is a very safe drug, although the side effects of headache, flushing, and dizziness can be disturbing to the patient. In this patient, the suspicion of angina pectoris due to arteriosclerotic heart disease should be relatively low, since the incidence of coronary artery disease in a 41-year-old (premenopausal) female is very low in the absence of other risk factors, and the history and treadmill test results are not suggestive of exertional angina. A trial of nitroglycerin, therefore, although safe, would probably not be that helpful as the next step in the diagnostic and therapeutic processes. A dramatic response of the chest pain to nitroglycerin may, however, suggest the presence of Prinzmetal's angina or esophageal spasm.

(2) The use of a beta-blocker drug may also be indicated as an early step in the diagnosis and treatment of chest pain. However, beta-blockers cannot be used in the same way as nitroglycerin to treat an acute attack and, in that sense, are less useful as a diagnostic test. Moreover, beta-blocker therapy is less specific than nitrate therapy and may be associated with more side effects. Beta-blockers also decrease the frequency and severity of chest pain associated with the mitral valve prolapse syndrome, which this patient could conceivably have. A reduction in chest pain, therefore, might be consistent with a diagnosis of either coronary artery disease or mitral valve prolapse syndrome. Furthermore, placing the patient on beta-blocker therapy may interfere with subsequent exercise testing (thallium or nuclear wall motion).

(3) A thallium stress test would be worthwhile as a diagnostic tool when either the history or routine electrocardiographic stress test is suggestive but nondiagnostic of coronary artery disease. This case fits this category, and a thallium stress test would be a logical choice. A negative test would be good evidence against the diagnosis of significant coronary artery disease and angina pectoris, while a positive test would be very strong evidence in favor of this diagnosis.

(4) Coronary fluoroscopy is a useful test when the diagnosis of coronary artery disease is being considered. It is a highly

specific although not very sensitive test in younger patients. Therefore, the absence of demonstrable coronary calcification in this patient would not be significant evidence against the diagnosis of coronary artery disease, while the presence of coronary calcification would be strong evidence for the existence of significant coronary disease. Coronary fluoroscopy is a simple noninvasive test do do, and its high specificity in younger patients makes it a useful test in this group.

(5) An echocardiogram (two-dimensional and M-mode) would be another worthwhile noninvasive test for a patient with chest pain and palpitations of uncertain etiology, especially if a systolic murmur and/or systolic click is heard. The demonstration of mitral valve prolapse on echocardiography might explain these symptoms in this patient. However, it should be kept in mind that since the presence of mitral valve prolapse on echocardiography is a relatively common finding in middle-aged females, the demonstration of this finding does not necessarily establish a cause-and-effect relationship for a given patient's symptoms, and does not exclude the coexistence of coronary artery disease or other organic heart disease in addition to the mitral valve prolapse syndrome.

PART B

Coronary fluoroscopy and thallium stress testing are both done, and both are negative. A two-dimensional and M-mode echocardiogram are performed next and show no evidence of mitral valve prolapse or other cardiac abnormalities. An empiric trial of nitroglycerin does seem to accelerate the relief of her chest pains, while a trial on propranolol has no apparent beneficial effect on preventing episodes of chest pain and appears to even have increased the frequency of pain. At this point you would:

1. Order an upper GI series
2. Order a nuclear wall motion exercise test
3. Order a Holter monitor
4. Start the patient on long-acting nitrates
5. Suggest cardiac catheterization and coronary arteriography

Discussion

(1) An upper GI series is often done as part of the workup of "atypical" chest pain, since several causes of chest pain which can mimic the pain of coronary origin can originate in the

gastrointestinal tract, such as (reflux) esophagitis, gastritis, peptic ulcer disease, and esophageal spasm. The latter can be further confused with coronary artery disease, since the associated chest pain often responds to nitrates and even to calcium blockers. It is a fallacy to assume that a demonstrated abnormality of the GI tract such as a hiatal hernia (with or without reflux) is necessarily the cause of a patient's symptoms. Certainly many patients have such abnormalities, which may be symptomatic or asymptomatic but may not necessarily be responsible for particular chest pain. In order to establish a reasonable cause-and-effect relationship of an abnormality of the upper GI tract to a particular chest pain, the history should be completely compatible with this etiology and there should be a careful search to exclude evidence of coexisting coronary artery disease. A therapeutic trial of antacids or a Bernstein test (infusion of dilute hydrochloric acid into the esophagus) as a provocative test may be useful to establish a causal relationship between gastroesophageal reflux and chest pain.

(2) An exercise wall motion test is helpful when the history, exercise electrocardiogram, and perhaps thallium stress tests are equivocal but nondiagnostic. A perfectly normal exercise wall motion test combined with a negative thallium stress test would be strong evidence against significant coronary artery disease. Since the patient's symptoms are not exercise related, however, this test may be less useful in this situation.

(3) A Holter monitor is often very helpful in patients with nonexertional chest pain, since it may detect symptomatic (as well as asymptomatic) episodes of ischemia by demonstration of ST segment depression or elevation. For most meaningful results, a two-channel system should be utilized which records two separate leads simultaneously from two separate areas of the heart (anterolateral and inferior), and the system should have a good frequency response in order to make ST segment changes interpretable. The absence of ST segment abnormalities during an episode of chest pain using this type of system is strong evidence against myocardial ischemia, while the occurrence of ST segment abnormalities with episodes of chest pain is of diagnostic value. This is especially useful in cases of resting or "Prinzmetal's" angina.

(4) Prophylactic empiric use of a long-acting nitrate is certainly an approach that could be taken at this point on the basis of the response to sublingual nitroglycerin and may result in partial or even complete relief of symptoms. However, this might still leave the diagnosis in question, and would probably not be the best approach in a patient of this age group in whom

more information is desirable for future management and for
advice on life-style, employment, and prognosis.

(5) Coronary arteriography is certainly the definitive test at
the present time for the presence of coronary artery disease,
and would be the most direct method of making this diagnosis.
Whether it should be done at this point in the work-up is de-
batable, since the previously discussed noninvasive tests,
depending upon the results, may obviate the need for this invasive study (or may provide more justification for doing it).
It should also be borne in mind that the demonstration of mild
to moderate coronary artery disease on arteriography does
not establish a cause and effect relationship to episodes of
chest pain, and objective evidence of ischemia as well as
coronary artery narrowing should be sought.

PART C

An upper GI series is done and is negative. An exercise wall
motion study is also totally normal. A Holter monitor is
ordered before considering coronary arteriography, and is
abnormal.   Figure 12-4A illustrates a strip obtained from the
Holter monitor when the patient is symptom-free.   Figure 12-4B
shows a strip taken shortly afterward when the patient first
complains of chest pain, and 12-4C is taken a few seconds later
with continued chest pain. The final strip (Figure 12-4D) is
taken with continued chest pain and development of palpitations.
After a few minutes, the patient takes a sublingual nitroglycerin
and the pain is relieved and the ECG changes seen on the Holter
monitor resolve. A diagnosis of Prinzmetal's angina is made
and coronary arteriography is recommended and done. The
angiogram is entirely normal. At this point, ergonovine is given
in small divided doses up to a total of 0.4 mg, at which point
the patient again has her characteristic chest pain and develops
ST segment elevations, most marked in the inferior electrocardiographic leads. A repeat coronary arteriogram now shows
complete obstruction of the mid-right coronary artery, and
100 mg of nitroglycerin is given directly into the right coronary
artery with return of the angiogram to normal and relief of the
chest pain and ST segment abnormalities (see Figure 6-4).

At this point you would:

1.   Recommend coronary artery bypass surgery
2.   Recommend percutaneous transluminal coronary angio-
     plasty (PTCA)
3.   Start the patient on a course of nitrates
4.   Start the patient on a course of calcium blocker drug

VI
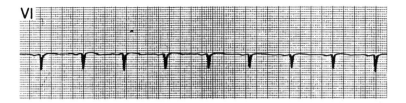

V5
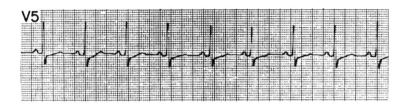

Figure 12-4A.

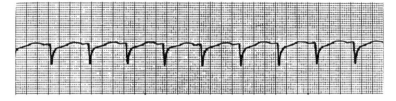

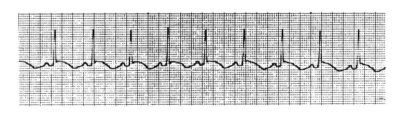

Figure 12-4B.

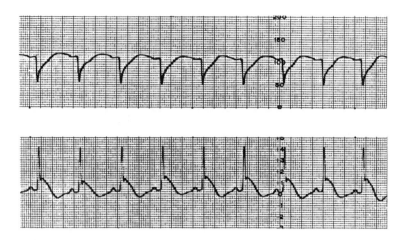

Figure 12-4C.

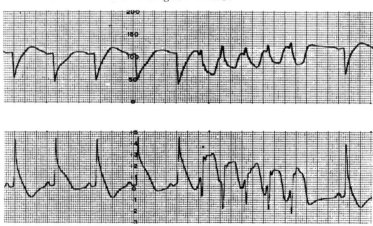

Figure 12-4D.

5. Both 3 and 4
6. Start the patient on a beta-blocker drug

Discussion

(1) This patient has documented coronary artery spasm responsible for her chest pain and fits into the category of Prinzmetal's
angina, with characteristic episodic ST segment elevation associated with chest pain and ventricular arrhythmias. Coronary
artery bypass surgery is contraindicated in the case of coronary
artery spasm without associated arteriosclerotic coronary
narrowing. It is recommended only when coronary artery spasm
occurs in conjunction with a significant arteriosclerotic lesion,
which often is the case. Patients with coronary artery spasm
demonstrated in one location can also have coronary artery
spasm elsewhere in the coronary artery tree at the same time
or subsequently in their course, and surgery would therefore
be not only unnecessary but also not helpful.
      (2) PTCA would likewise be contraindicated in coronary ar-
tery spasm with normal coronary arteries. There is an increased
incidence of restenosis at the site of angioplasty when arteriosclerotic lesions associated with coronary artery spasm are
dilated, and therefore this is not a recommended mode of therapy
in this setting.
      (3) Nitrates are usually highly effective in the treatment and
prevention of coronary artery spasm, especially when used in
higher doses. Long-acting nitrates would certainly be one of
the treatments of choice in a patient with Prinzmetal's angina
and may be the only treatment necessary.
      (4) Calcium channel blocking drugs are extremely effective in
the treatment of coronary artery spasm and are probably at
least as effective if not more effective than nitrates. Any of the
three available drugs—nifedipine, diltiazem, or verapamil—
may be used, with nifedipine and diltiazem having somewhat
more effect on coronary vasodilatation than verapamil.
      (5) A combination of a nitrate and a calcium channel blocking
drug is the most effective treatment for this disorder. Ordinarily, one or the other drug would be initiated alone, since either
may be completely effective. If maximal necessary dosage of
either drug is not totally effective or is not tolerated, combination therapy is usually successful in preventing chest pain.
      (6) Beta-blocker drugs are relatively contraindicated for
Prinzmetal's angina, since they increase rather than decrease
coronary artery tone, and may therefore increase the tendency
for spasm. The one exception is the occurrence of Prinzmetal's
angina in conjunction with fixed arteriosclerotic lesions, in

which case a reduction of myocardial oxygen consumption by use of a beta-blocker drug would be beneficial when combined with a nitrate, calcium channel blocker, or both.

PART D

The patient is started on a long-acting nitrate with considerable but incomplete relief of her symptoms. A calcium channel blocking drug is added, with total prevention of episodes of chest pain. Her repeat Holter is entirely normal without any ST segment abnormalities or arrhythmias.

DISCUSSION OF CASE 4

This case illustrates a fairly typical case of Prinzmetal's (variant) angina due to coronary artery spasm and illustrates the usual results of workup and treatment. A treadmill exercise test can be negative, positive, or equivocal in this disease, and other tests usually diagnostic of coronary artery disease such as thallium and exercise wall motion may be entirely normal. A Holter monitor (or in-hospital monitoring) is usually the most effective way of establishing the correct diagnosis. If coronary artery spasm is suspected either on the basis of the history or the electrocardiogram, coronary arteriography is indicated to rule out the presence of a combination of a fixed lesion with an additional component of spasm, or transient occlusion which may require coronary artery bypass surgery. If the coronary arteriogram is normal, ergonovine is then given (with intracoronary nitroglycerin available) with continuous electrocardiographic and arterial pressure monitoring to demonstrate evocable spasm in either the left or right coronary artery system. Prinzmetal's angina is often associated with ventricular arrhythmias and conduction abnormalities, and symptoms resulting from these occurrences may be present in addition to (or instead of) chest pain.

Index